Pharmacology for Pharmacy and the Health Sciences

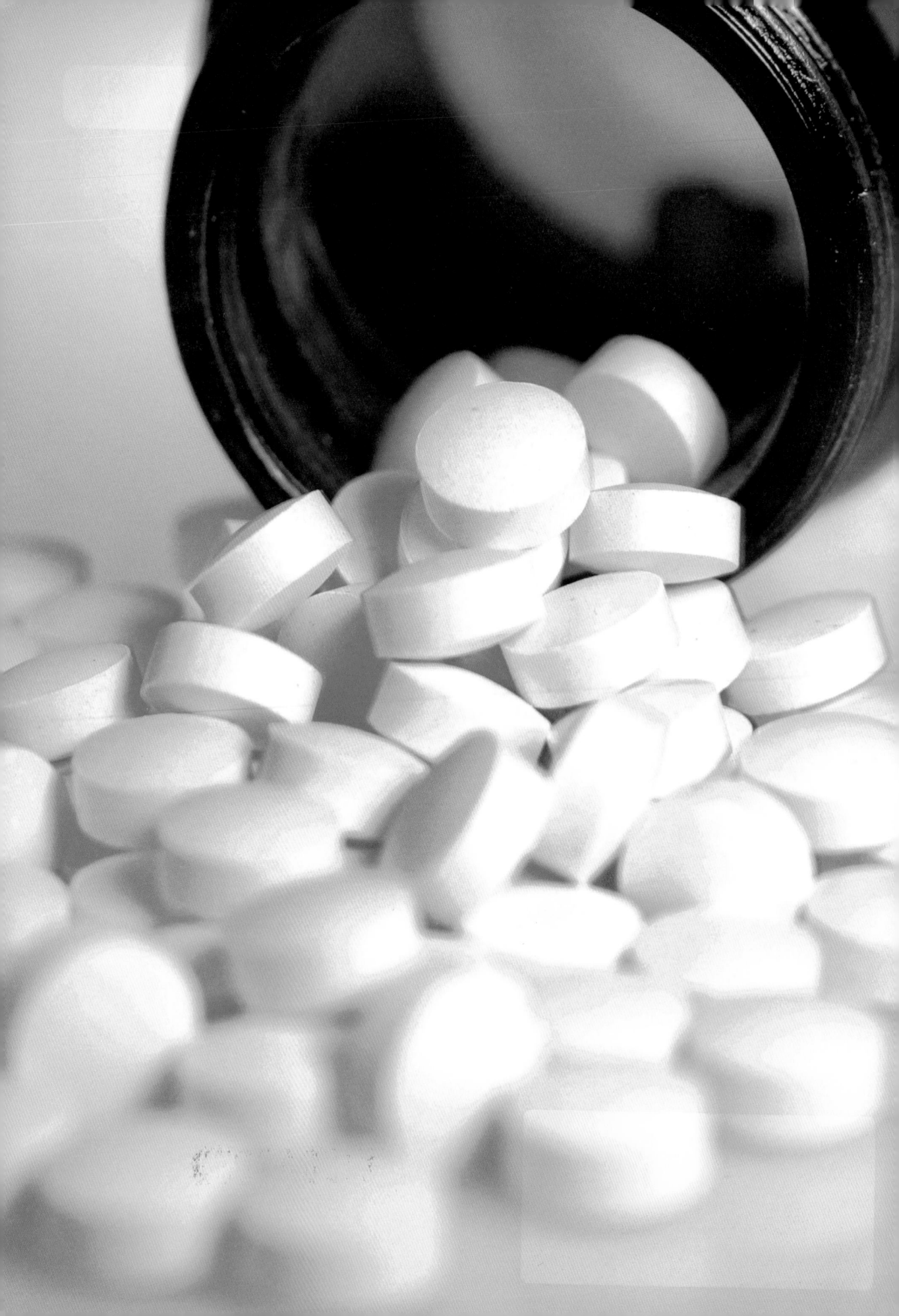

Pharmacology for Pharmacy and the Health Sciences

A patient-centred approach

Second edition

Michael Boarder

Formerly Professor of Pharmacology, Leicester School of Pharmacy,
De Montfort University, UK

Jane Dixon

Senior Lecturer, Leicester School of Pharmacy, De Montfort University, UK

David Newby

Associate Professor, Discipline of Clinical Pharmacology,
School of Medicine and Public Health, University of Newcastle, Australia

Phyllis Navti

Divisional Lead Prescribing Advisor, Leicestershire County and
Rutland Primary Care Trust NHS, and Senior Lecturer in Pharmacy Practice,
Leicester School of Pharmacy, De Montfort University, UK

Tyra Zetterström

Reader in Neuropharmacology, Leicester School of Pharmacy,
De Montfort University, UK

OXFORD
UNIVERSITY PRESS

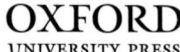

OXFORD
UNIVERSITY PRESS

Great Clarendon Street, Oxford, OX2 6DP,
United Kingdom

Oxford University Press is a department of the University of Oxford.
It furthers the University's objective of excellence in research, scholarship,
and education by publishing worldwide. Oxford is a registered trade mark of
Oxford University Press in the UK and in certain other countries

First Edition 2010

Impression: 1

Published in the United States of America by Oxford University Press
198 Madison Avenue, New York, NY 10016, United States of America

British Library Cataloguing in Publication Data

Data available

Library of Congress Control Number: 2016951219

ISBN 978-0-19-872883-2

Printed in Great Britain by
Bell & Bain Ltd., Glasgow

Acknowledgements

We would like to thank all those involved in the first edition of this book, and extend our special thanks to a number of individuals who have been particularly helpful with this second edition. Those people are: Benjamin Gronier (for help with Chapters 14 and 15); Laura Smith (for help with Chapter 22); Amanda Kemp (for material in the workbooks in Chapters 20 and 21); Anisha Patel (for material in the workbooks in Part 1); Geoff Hall (for his expertise in areas of medicinal chemistry); and Peter Dixon (for his unerring attention to detail).

Contents at a glance

Contents in full

Abbreviations

5′-dFCyd	5′-deoxy-5′-fluorocytidine		ARC	arcuate nucleus
5′-dFUrd	5′-deoxy-5′-fluorouridine		AT-III	antithrombin-III
5-ASA	5-aminosalicylic acid		ATP	adenosine triphosphate
5-FU	5-fluorouracil		ATRA	all-trans retinoic acid
5-HT	5-hydroxytryptamine (serotonin)		AV	atrioventricular
5-HTT	serotonin 5-HT transporter		AWS	alcohol withdrawal syndrome
6-MP	6-mercaptopurine		BAC	blood alcohol content/concentration
6-MMP	6-methylmercaptopurine		BCR	breakpoint cluster region
6-MTG	6-methylthioguanine		BDNF	brain-derived neurotrophic factor
6-MTIMP	6-methylthioinosine monophosphate		bFGF	basic fibroblast growth factor
6-MTITP	6-methylthioinosine triphosphate		BMI	body mass index
6-TG	6-thioguanine		BP	blood pressure
6-TGMP	6-thioguanine monophosphate		BPH	benign prostatic hyperplasia
6-TGTP	6-thioguanine triphosphate		cAMP	cyclic adenosine monophosphate
6-TIMP	6-thioinosine monophosphate		CaM	calmodulin
6-TUA	6-thiouric acid		CB_1	endogenous cannabinoid receptor 1
6-TXMP	6-thioxanthosine monophosphate		CB_2	endogenous cannabinoid receptor 2
A&E	Accident and Emergency		CBT	cognitive behavioural therapy
A2RA (AIIRA)	angiotensin II receptor antagonist		CCK	cholecystokinin
A ß	amyloid-ß-peptides		CCU	coronary care unit
ACE	angiotensin-converting enzyme		CD	cluster of differentiation, cytidine deaminase
ACh	acetylcholine			
AChR	acetylcholine receptor		CDC	Centers for Disease Control and Prevention, complement-dependent cytotoxicity
ACS	acute coronary syndrome			
ACTH	adrenocorticotrophic hormone			
ADCC	antibody-dependent cellular cytotoxicity		CDK	cyclin-dependent kinase
ADH	antidiuretic hormone		CES	carboxylesterase
ADHD	attention deficit hyperactivity disorder		CL	corpus luteum
ADME	absorption, distribution, metabolism, elimination		CMF	cyclophosphamide, methotrexate, and fluorouracil
			CML	chronic myeloid leukaemia
ADP	adenosine diphosphate		CMV	cytomegalovirus
AED	antiepileptic drug		CNS	central nervous system
AF	atrial fibrillation		CO	cardiac output
AgRP	agouti-related protein		COMT	catechol-O-methyltransferase
AIC	5-aminoimidazole-4-carboxamide		COPD	chronic obstructive pulmonary disease
ALL	acute lymphoblastic leukaemia		CORB	confusion, oxygen, respiratory rate, blood pressure
AML	acute myeloid leukaemia			
AMP	adenosine monophosphate		COX	cyclo-oxygenase
AMPA	α-amino-3-hydroxy-5-methyl-4-isoxazolepropionic acid		CRH	corticotrophin releasing hormone
			CRP	C-reactive protein
AMPK	AMP-activated protein kinase		CSM	Committee on Safety of Medicines
ANS	autonomic nervous system		CTPA	computed tomography pulmonary angiography
APC	antigen-presenting cell			
APML	acute promyelocytic leukaemia		CTZ	chemoreceptor trigger zone
aPTT	activated partial thromboplastin time		CV	cardiovascular
ARB	angiotensin receptor blocker			

CVD	cardiovascular disease		GMAWS	Glasgow Modified Alcohol Withdrawal Scale
CYP450	cytochrome P450		GMP	guanosine monophosphate
DAG	diacylglycerol		GMPS	guanosine monophosphate synthetase
DAT	dopamine transporter		GnRH	gonadotropin-releasing hormone
dCMP	deoxycytidine monophosphate		GORD	gastro-oesophageal reflux disease
dCTP	deoxycytidine triphosphate		GPCR	G-protein-coupled receptor
DDC	dopa-decarboxylase		GRE	glucocorticoid-responsive element
DHFR	dihydrofolate reductase		GTI	gastrointestinal tract infection
DIT	diiodotyrosine		GTN	glyceryl trinitrate
DMARD	disease-modifying anti-rheumatic drug		GTP	guanosine triphosphate
DMT	dimethyltryptamine		Hb	haemoglobin
DP	diphosphate		HCV	hepatitis C virus
DPK	diphosphate kinase		HDAC	histone deacetylase
DPP-4	dipeptidyl peptidase 4		HDL	high density lipoprotein
DT	delirium tremens		HER1	human epidermal growth factor receptor 1
DTIC	dacarbazine		HER2	human epidermal growth factor receptor 2
dTMP	2′-deoxythymidylate monophosphate		HIF-1a	hypoxia-inducible factor 1a
dUMP	2′-deoxyuridylate monophosphate		HIT	heparin-induced thrombocytopenia
DVT	deep vein thrombosis		HMG	hydroxymethylglutaryl
EC_{50}	concentration giving 50% of maximum response		HPA	hypothalamic–pituitary–adrenal
ECG	electrocardiogram		HPRT	hypoxanthine phosphoribosyl transferase
ECL	enterochromaffin-like		HR	heart rate
EDRF	endothelium-derived relaxing factor		HSD	hydroxysteroid dehydrogenase
EDV	end diastolic volume		HSV	herpes simplex virus
EEG	electroencephalogram		HTA	histone acetyltransferase
EGFR	epidermal growth factor receptor		IBD	inflammatory bowel disease
ERCC1	excision repair cross-complementing protein		IBS	irritable bowel syndrome
ERK	extracellular signal-regulated kinase		IBS-A	irritable bowel syndrome—alternating diarrhoea and constipation
FBC	full blood count		IBS-C	irritable bowel syndrome—constipation dominant
FdUDP	fluorodeoxyuridylate diphosphate		IBS-D	irritable bowel syndrome—diarrhoea dominant
FdUMP	fluorodeoxyuridylate monophosphate		IBS-M	irritable bowel syndrome—mixed diarrhoea and constipation
FdUTP	fluorodeoxyuridylate triphosphate		ICAM-1	intercellular adhesion molecule 1
FEV_1	forced expiratory volume in one second		ICD-10	International Statistical Classification of Diseases and Related Health Problems, 10th revision
FSH	follicle-stimulating hormone		IFL	irinotecan, fluorouracil, and leucovorin
FUDP	fluorouracil diphosphate		Ig	immunoglobulin
FUMP	fluorouracil monophosphate		IGF-1	insulin-like growth factor 1
FUTP	fluorouracil triphosphate		IL	interleukin
FVC	forced vital capacity		IMPD	inosine monophosphate dehydrogenase
GABA	gamma-aminobutyric acid		INR	International Normalized Ratio
G-CSF	granulocyte colony stimulating factor		IP_3	inositol trisphosphate
GDNF	glial cell line derived neurotrophic factor		IRS	insulin-receptor substrate
GDP	guanosine diphosphate		ISCD	Independent Scientific Committee on Drugs
GH	growth hormone		JAK	Janus kinase
GHRH	growth hormone releasing hormone			
GI	gastrointestinal			
GINA	Global Initiative for Asthma			
GIP	glucose-dependent insulinotropic peptide			
GLP-1	glucagon-like peptide-1			
GLUT-2	glucose transporter 2			
GLUT-4	glucose transporter 4			

K_D	dissociation constant (a measure of the affinity of a ligand for its receptor)
LABA	long-acting selective β_2-adrenoceptor agonist
LAMA	long-acting muscarinic antagonist
LDL	low density lipoprotein
LFT	liver function test
LH	luteinizing hormone
LHA	lateral hypothalamic area
LH-RH	luteinizing hormone-releasing hormone
LMWH	low molecular weight heparin
LSD	lysergic acid diethylamide
LV	left ventricle
LVEF	left ventricular ejection fraction
MAC	*Mycobacterium avium* complex
mAChR	muscarinic acetylcholine receptor
MAO	monoamine oxidase
MAPK	mitogen-activated protein kinase
MDI	metered dose inhaler
MDMA	3,4-methylenedioxymetamphetamine (ecstasy)
MEG	magnetoencephalography
MDT	multidisciplinary team
MHC	major histocompatibility complex
MHRA	Medicines and Healthcare Products Regulatory Agency
MI	myocardial infarction
MIT	monoiodotyrosine
MLCK	myosin light chain kinase
MLCP	myosin light chain phosphatase
mLDL	modified LDL
MMP	matrix metalloproteinases
MP	monophosphate
MPK	monophosphate kinase
MRI	magnetic resonance imaging
mRNA	messenger ribonucleic acid
MRSA	meticillin-resistant *Staphylococcus aureus*
MS	multiple sclerosis
MSH	melanocyte stimulating hormone
MTIC	methyltriazenyl-imidazole-carboxamide
mTOR	mammalian target of rapamycin
NA	noradrenaline (norepinephrine)
nAChR	nicotinic acetylcholine receptor
NADPH	nicotinamide adenine dinucleotide phosphate
NARI	selective noradrenaline reuptake inhibitor
NARTI	nucleoside analogue reverse transcriptase inhibitor
NaSSA	noradrenergic and specific serotonergic antidepressant
NDP	nucleoside diphosphate
NFAT	nuclear factor of activated T-cells
NF-κB	nuclear factor kappa-light-chain-enhancer of activated B-cells
NICE	National Institute of Health and Care Excellence
NK	natural killer
NK-1	neurokinin 1
NMDA	*N*-methyl-D-aspartate
NNRTI	non-nucleoside reverse transcriptase inhibitor
NO	nitric oxide
NOAC	novel oral anticoagulants
NOP	nociceptin/orphanin
NPY	neuropeptide Y
NSAID	non-steroidal anti-inflammatory drug
NSCLC	non-small-cell lung cancer
NSTEMI	non-ST-segment elevation myocardial infarction
NtARTI	nucleotide analogue reverse transcriptase inhibitor
ORS	oral rehydration solution
PAE	post-antibiotic effect
PAF	platelet-activating factor
PAG	periaqueductal grey
PAI-1	plasminogen activator inhibitor 1
PAI-2	plasminogen activator inhibitor 2
PAR	platelet thrombin receptor
PCA	patient-controlled analgesia
PCI	percutaneous coronary intervention
PCP	phencyclidine
PCP	*Pneumocystis jiroveci (carinii)* pneumonia
PDE	phosphodiesterase
PDGFR	platelet-derived growth factor receptor
PE	pulmonary embolism
PEF	peak expiratory flow
PEG	polyethylene glycol
PET	positron emission tomography
PGE_1	prostaglandin E_1
PGE_2	prostaglandin E_2
PGI_2	prostaglandin I_2 (prostacyclin)
PI	protease inhibitor
PI3K	phosphoinositide 3-kinase
PIP_2	phosphatidylinositol bisphosphate
PKA	protein kinase A
PKC	protein kinase C
PLA_2	phospholipase A_2
PLC	phospholipase C
PMA	para-methoxyamphetamine
PML	promyelocytic leukaemia gene
PP	pancreatic polypeptide
PPARγ	peroxisome proliferator activator receptor gamma

PPI	proton pump inhibitor
PSI	pneumonia severity index
PUVA	psoralen + UVA treatment
PVN	paraventricular nucleus
QRS	QRS complex on an electrocardiogram
QT	QT segment on an electrocardiogram
RA	rheumatoid arthritis
RAAS	renin–angiotensin–aldosterone system
RANKL	receptor activator of nuclear factor $\kappa\beta$ ligand
RBC	red blood cell
RF	rheumatoid factor
rRNA	ribosomal RNA
RSV	respiratory syncytial virus
RTI	respiratory tract infection, reverse transcriptase inhibitor
RXR	retinoid X receptor
SA	sinoatrial node
SABA	short-acting selective β_2-adrenoceptor agonist
SAMA	short-acting muscarinic antagonist
SE	status epilepticus
SERM	selective oestrogen receptor modulator
SERT	serotonin (5-HT) transporter
SGLT	sodium–glucose co-transporter
SIADH	syndrome of inappropriate antidiuretic hormone
SNRI	serotonin and noradrenaline reuptake inhibitor
SSRI	selective serotonin reuptake inhibitor
STAT	signal transducers and activators of transcription
STEMI	ST-segment elevation myocardial infarction
STI	sexually transmitted infection
SV	stroke volume
T_3	triiodothyronine
T_4	tetraiodothyronine (thyroxine)
TB	tuberculosis
TC	total plasma cholesterol
TCA	tricyclic antidepressant
TCR	T-cell receptor
TDM	therapeutic drug monitoring
TENS	transcutaneous electrical stimulation

THC	tetrahydrocannabinol
Th1	T-helper 1 cell
Th2	T-helper 2 cell
ThioTEPA	N,N',N''-triethylenethiophosphoramide
TNF	tumour necrosis factor
TNF-α	tumour necrosis factor alpha
TNM	T, extent of the tumour; N, number of lymph nodes involved; M, presence of metastasis
TP	thymidine phosphorylase, triphosphate
tPA	tissue plasminogen activator
TPMT	thiopurine-S-methyl transferase
TPR	total peripheral resistance
TR	thyroid receptor
TRH	thyrotrophin-releasing hormone
tRNA	transfer RNA
TRP	transient receptor potential
TS	thymidylate synthetase
TSH	thyroid-stimulating hormone
TXA$_2$	thromboxane A$_2$
UA/NSTEMI	unstable angina, non-ST-segment elevation myocardial infarction
UDP	uridine diphosphate
UFH	unfractionated heparin
UGT	uridine diphosphate glucuronyltransferase
ULABA	ultra-long acting β_2-adrenoceptor agonist
UTI	urinary tract infection
UV	ultraviolet
UVA	ultraviolet A
UVB	ultraviolet B
VCAM-1	vascular cell adhesion molecule 1
VEGF	vascular endothelial growth factor
VEGF-A	vascular endothelial growth factor A
VIP	vasoactive intestinal peptide
VLDL	very low density lipoprotein
VMH	ventromedial hypothalamic nucleus
VTA	ventral tegmental area
VTE	venous thromboembolism
WBC	white blood cell
WCC	white cell count
WE	Wernicke's encephalopathy
WHO	World Health Organization
XO	xanthine oxidase

Clinical clerking abbreviations

PC	Presenting complaint		DS	Drug sensitivities
HPC	History of presenting complaint		O/E	On examination
PMH	Past medical history		FH	Family history
SH	Social history		O/Q	On questioning
DH	Drug history		O/O	On observation

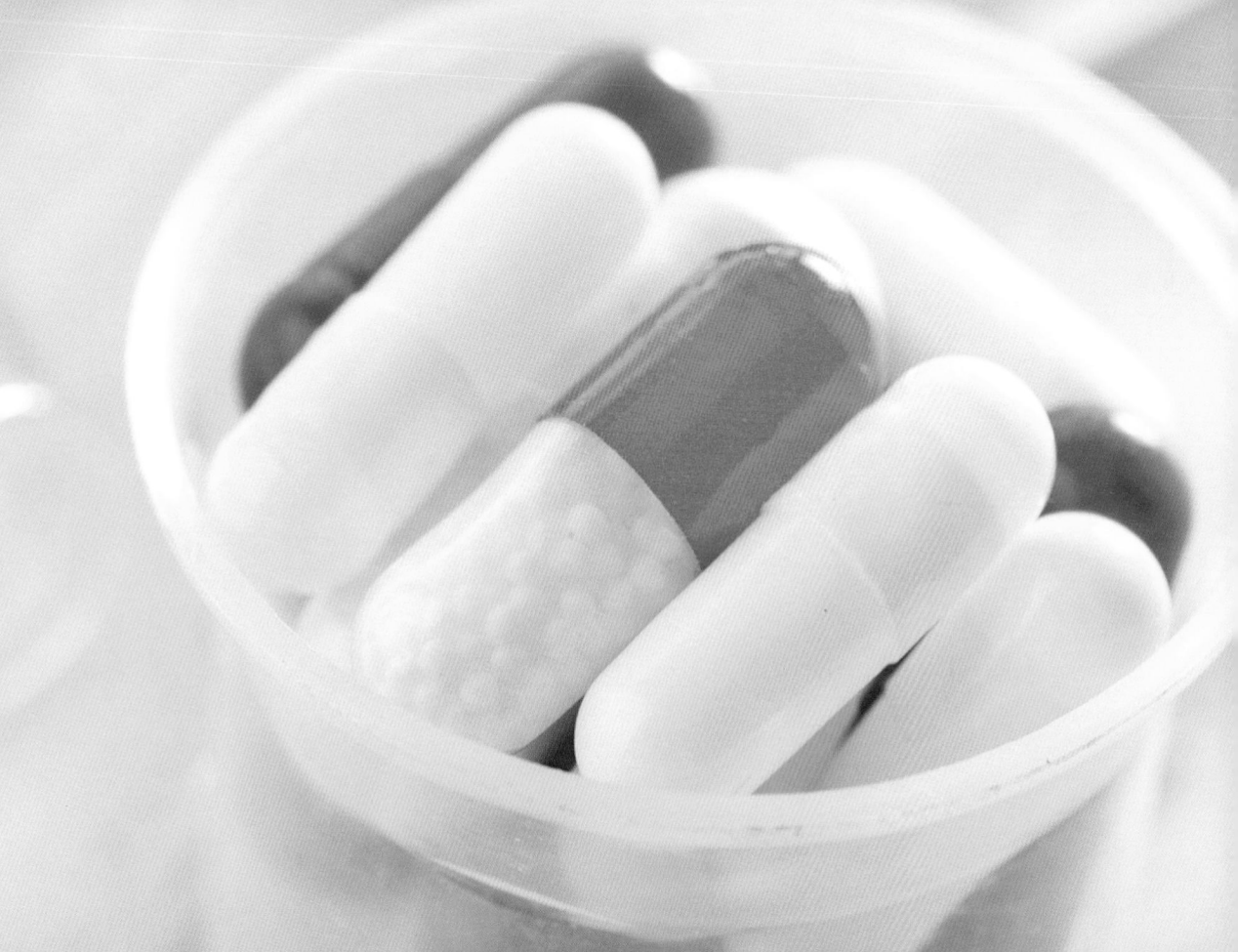

Part 1
Introduction

Chapter 1
Drugs, patients, and this book

Pharmacology—*a **patient-centred** approach?* What does this mean? Let's start with a patient.

> It's morning. Gerald is in his own home, sitting hunched in his chair, talking in a quiet monotone, without movement of his mask-like face, his hands trembling, but otherwise still. He doesn't get up to greet you, doesn't reach out to shake your hand. It's not that he can't do these things, but they are difficult for him; sometimes he doesn't know whether he can do them or not. Two patches of cells in his brain have died, and this means that his brain cannot plan movements and control his body. He takes his medication—it's not easy: his hands are shaking, swallowing is difficult. Half an hour later he stands, upright and confident, moves across the room normally, and now he reaches out to shake your hand firmly, smiling and chatting.[1]

We want you to be able to understand the various aspects of this situation.

1) What is wrong with the patient in the first place. **We need to understand this at the cellular and molecular level** if we are to understand the action of drugs.

2) The main drug treatments that are used to treat or manage the condition to benefit the patient.

3) **How drugs work at the cellular and molecular level to benefit the patient**. This is where you really *understand* how drugs help people.

This book is written on the basis that understanding the patient's response to drugs and the cellular and molecular basis of drug treatment are the same thing.

When you look at our patient Gerald, see his initial disability, and then watch how the drugs change him, you should be able to picture in your mind what is happening in his brain; how the drug is entering his brain and changing the way it works. As a result you will understand what the strengths and weaknesses of his treatment are, and what the future holds for him. You will also be in a good position to understand new drugs and approaches to treatment as they are introduced in the future.

We introduce our patients as individuals. We tell stories around them so that you will think of them as individuals. They are people, like you and me, our mums and dads, our children. They *are* you and me. **Pharmacology is about people**.

1.1 How does this fit in with your career development in the changing world of healthcare delivery?

The need for this book stems from the likely nature of healthcare delivery in the future. Changes to this are under way, driven by governments, professional bodies, and healthcare professionals themselves. In a number of countries, pharmacists are expected to play a greater role in healthcare delivery in the future: pharmacists are

expected to become more **patient-centred**, with both pharmacists and nurses playing a primary role in prescribing drugs in many healthcare settings.

As Patrick Vallance and Trevor Smart wrote in the *British Journal of Pharmacology*:[2]

---

1 Gerald's illness and its treatment are explored in Chapter 17.

2 Vallance P, Smart T. The future of pharmacology. *British Journal of Pharmacology* 2006; 147 (Suppl 1): S304–S307.

Prescribers are changing. Getting onto the register to practice as a doctor brings rather few specific rights. In fact just about the only one is the right to prescribe medicines. However, nurses and pharmacists are also gaining these rights and this trend seems unlikely to reverse. Indeed, it makes sense to broaden the range of prescribers, and the challenge will be to ensure an appropriate pharmacological underpinning to ensure safe and effective use of medicines.

This book will prepare you for these future challenges.

1.2   So, what is pharmacology?

Firstly, **pharmacology is a science**, so be prepared to learn a lot of science in this book. And be prepared to refer back to your basic biology, to refresh your memory about systems in the body—the heart and circulation, digestive system, the nervous system, etc. After all, it is these that go wrong when we get ill, so it is these that we will discuss as we go through medical conditions and their treatment.

Pharmacology is a broad science, running from the chemistry of drugs, through their physiological effect, to treatment of the sick. In 1968, in the book *Principles of Drug Action*, Avram Goldstein and colleagues defined it as follows:

> Pharmacology is the science of drugs, their chemical constitution, their biologic action, and their therapeutic application in man.

Today, molecular and cell biology are at the heart of pharmacology—drugs are molecules, and they interact with other molecules inside us. This changes cells, organ systems, and eventually our bodies and our minds, for good or for bad.

The molecules with which drugs interact are often, but not always, proteins in our cells. The composition of the protein assemblies within our cells is initially defined by what we inherit from our parents—our genome. It's not surprising then that modern pharmacology is dependent on the understanding and techniques of molecular biology and genomics. This is where future advances, the nature of which we can only guess at, will have their beginnings. This is not an academic exercise—it is at the heart of drug discovery in the pharmaceutical industry, and the treatment of illnesses.

1.3   How to use this book

The chapters in this book are divided into six parts. Those in the first part, following this Introduction, deal with how drugs act to change the body (Chapter 2) and what happens to the drug itself after it has entered the body (Chapter 3). The remaining chapters are concerned with clinical topics, starting with thromboembolic disorders, ending with cancers, and on the way dealing with such common conditions as heart attacks, asthma, epilepsy, depression, and infections.

All of the following chapters have **boxes**, separated from the main text, which develop subjects and issues in greater detail. In some cases this is a more in-depth treatment of the science; in others it is a further exploration of clinical issues.

The clinically oriented chapters, in Parts 2–6, end with **workbooks**, which can be downloaded as detailed below. Here this book takes on an unusual aspect.

Fictional characters appear in a storyline in these workbooks; some of them become ill and are admitted to hospital. The patient's details and clinical history are presented in a **clinical clerking** format. The medical staff treating them are introduced into the narrative, and the patient's diagnosis is made on the basis of the clinical clerking. A treatment plan is devised, and the workbook follows the progress of the fictional patients, mainly with respect to their medical condition, but also looking at the impact this has on their lives. The narratives are simple and are intended to graphically illustrate the individual nature of patient care. In many of the workbooks the same, or related, characters appear as their stories are developed.

From the point at which the diagnosis is made the workbooks have a further feature: questions designed to test your understanding of the clinical topic, of the science underpinning the drugs, and of the drug treatments themselves. By completing these workbooks, you will not only have been taken through the subject in an interactive manner, probing and developing your understanding of the subject, but will also have created a learning resource for yourself.

The material required to answer the questions is provided in the main text (and boxes) in the relevant chapter. In this sense each chapter is self-contained. In order to approach much of the material in these chapters, though, it is first necessary to understand the fundamental aspects of drug action and drug use, as explained in Chapters 2 and 3. For example, you need to understand the term 'antagonist', and to have a picture of how the body handles drugs introduced by different routes. Once

you are confident in your understanding of basic pharmacology, the clinical subjects pursued in the remainder of the book can be approached in any order.

In addition to the main text, boxes, and workbooks, you will find that each chapter begins with a list of definitions of **key terms** of particular relevance to the current topic. The clinical chapters end with a **drug summary table**—a quick reference source of the principal drugs used in each area, to which you can refer across, and within, chapters.

Some suggestions for **further reading** are provided at the end of each chapter, with examples exploring the basic science as well as the clinical application of pharmacology.

1.4 Comment for instructors

This book, with the feature of workbooks with narrative based around fictional characters, arose out of our experience of moving towards teaching patient-centred pharmacology to pharmacy students. The workbooks present in this text have their origin in those used in our teaching. They form the activity in small-group teaching sessions, each of which is preceded by a series of lectures covering the subject of the workbook. Here we have revised and extended the breadth of subjects covered in

the workbooks. In our strong emphasis on patients, we have strived to integrate the scientific basis of therapeutics with the clinical material. Our objective is that the science and the individual's therapeutic response are not seen as sequential (or, even worse, separate) material, but as a single integrated subject. We hope that you find this book interesting, but mostly we hope that it enthuses your students, motivating them to truly understand the pharmacological basis of therapeutics.

1.5 Online Resource Centre

Pharmacology for Pharmacy and the Health Sciences doesn't end with this printed book. Further materials are also available in the book's Online Resource Centre at www.oxfordtextbooks.co.uk/orc/boarder2e/.

The Online Resource Centre includes the following material for registered adopters of the book:

- **figures from the book** in electronic format, ready to download
- all **workbooks** included in this book in pdf format, for use in teaching seminars, workshops, etc.
- **suggested answers** to the questions posed in the workbooks.

⊙ Key references and suggested reading

Australian Prescriber. http://www.australianprescriber.com.

National Institute for Health and Care Excellence (NICE). http://www.nice.org.uk/.

Rossi S. (ed.). *Australian Medicines Handbook*. Adelaide: Australian Medicines Handbook Pty Ltd, 2016.

British National Formulary. London: Pharmaceutical Press, 2008.

Lexi-COMP online. http://www.lexi.com/.

Rote Liste. http://www.rote-liste.de/.

med-news: Medizinische Informationen für Ärzte und Apotheker. http://www.gfi-online.de/.

Chapter 2
How do drugs work?
An introduction

The drugs we are mainly interested in are those used to treat illnesses (therapeutic drugs). The majority (although not all) of these drugs are small molecules prepared by pharmaceutical companies, and our objective in this chapter is to provide an overview of how these drugs change bodily function. These principles of drug action will be encountered again and again in the medical use of the drugs that are discussed in the rest of this book. We consider here the most commonly encountered forms of drug action—there are other modes of action of drugs used in the clinic that we do not discuss in this chapter. Some are explained later.

To begin thinking about how drugs act we can note the following points.

1) Most drugs act at cellular targets, but some do act outside cells. The simplest example of this is the treatment of acid indigestion with bicarbonate. The stomach contains hydrochloric acid, giving it a very low pH. When this causes discomfort, bicarbonate can be used to increase the stomach's pH by neutralizing some of the acid. This occurs in the lumen of the stomach outside any cells. Examples of non-cellular targets are also found in drugs acting at proteins in the soluble part of the blood (the plasma). For instance, in Chapter 4 we will encounter drugs interacting with plasma enzymes that are required for blood clotting. These enzymes (the clotting factors) are inhibited by drugs such as heparin. Biological agents useful in tackling inflammatory diseases such as rheumatoid arthritis also have non-cellular targets. In this case they are directed against the mediators of inflammation such as the cytokine tumour necrosis factor-α. Many such agents are genetically engineered monoclonal antibodies that are long-lived in the blood, from where they interact with their targets.

2) The large majority of drug targets are proteins (Box 2.1). Clotting factors are proteins, but are unusual in that they are not cellular. The more usual cellular target proteins can be at the surface of the cell, or inside it (intracellular).

Box 2.1

Targets of drugs are mostly proteins

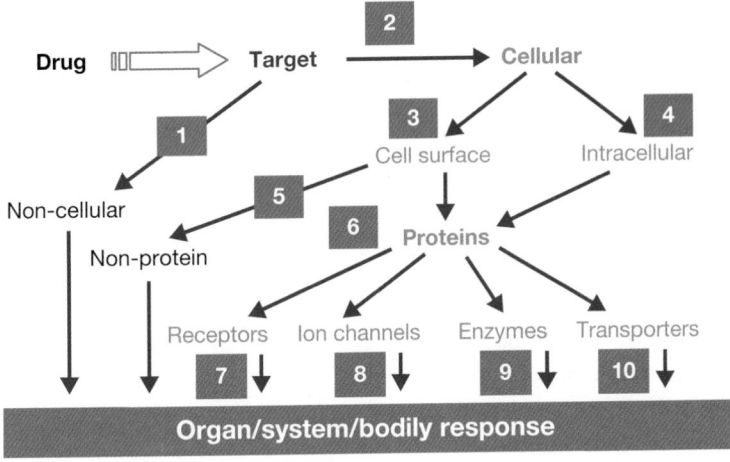

Figure a Drug targets

When a drug is administered it interacts with an initial target, the main classes of which are numbered on the scheme in Figure a.

1. A small minority of drugs interact with targets in the extracellular compartment.

2. The vast majority of drugs interact directly with molecules that are part of cells.

3. Some of these molecules are on the cell surface. This means that drugs that cannot enter cells (i.e. cannot pass through the lipid cell membrane because they are not lipid-soluble) can bind to this membrane component and change the function of the cell.

4. Lipophilic molecules, however, are able to cross the cell membrane and therefore have intracellular targets.

5. Some of the cell surface interactions are not with proteins, but with the lipid cell membrane itself. This type of interaction may contribute to the response to inhaled general anaesthetics,

although the action of such drugs is increasingly believed to derive from alterations to cell membrane proteins, such as ion channels.

6. Most of the interactions of drugs are with proteins, which may be on the cell surface or inside the cell. If the target protein is inside the cell, the drug must be able to pass through the cell membrane to reach it.

7. Receptors are the most common type of protein drug target, and can be either at the cell surface (usually intrinsic membrane proteins) or within the cell itself.

8–10. Other common types of protein target are ion channels, enzymes, or transporter proteins.

In this chapter we review the nature of drug action at these four main protein targets: receptors, ion channels, enzymes, and transporter proteins.

3) The majority of protein targets are receptors:[1] These are often cell surface receptors, for example those for adrenaline (epinephrine). In many cases, though, for example the targets for steroid drugs, the receptors are intracellular.

---

1 The term 'receptor' is sometimes used to mean the molecule, or part of a molecule, that a drug interacts with to have its effect. This would mean that all molecular targets of drugs are receptors. This is not how the term is used in this book. Here a receptor is taken to mean the molecule (usually a protein) that naturally occurring biological mediators (e.g. neurotransmitters, hormones, local mediators) bind to have their effect. This distinguishes receptors from enzymes, ion channels, transporters, or other proteins, which are all molecular targets for drug action, as set out in Box 2.1.

8

Chapter 2 How do drugs work? An introduction

4) Apart from receptors the most common protein targets for drugs are:

- **ion channels:** mainly on the cell surface, such as those targeted by calcium channel blockers used to lower blood pressure (Chapter 5)
- **enzymes:** mainly intracellular, as enzyme substrates (e.g. levodopa used to treat Parkinson's disease; Chapter 17) or inhibitors (e.g. ACE inhibitors used in the treatment of hypertension; Chapter 5)
- **transport proteins:** mainly cell surface, such as the transporters for neurotransmitters in the brain inhibited by SSRI-like drugs used to treat depression (Chapter 19).

2.1 Agonists and antagonists: drugs acting at receptors

Receptors have complex three-dimensional structures, within which pockets are formed that can be occupied by small molecules—either neurotransmitters, hormones, etc. produced by the body, or drugs. Such molecules are collectively referred to as **ligands** and they **bind** to specific sites on receptors. When bound they are said to **occupy** the receptors. Some (nearly all natural ligands, and some drugs) then **activate** the receptor to bring about changes to the cell where they are found. Ligands (both natural and drugs) which activate receptors are called **agonists**. Some ligands, however, bind but do not activate the receptor; these are **antagonists**. They have an effect because, by occupying receptors, they reduce the binding of the natural agonist, whose effect is thereby diminished. The general situation is illustrated in Figure 2.1 which

depicts events at a cell surface receptor in the presence of an agonist, an antagonist, or a combination of both.

2.1.1 Both agonists and antagonists are important in therapeutics

To help understand the principles of agonist and antagonist action we can consider adrenaline (epinephrine), a hormone secreted from the adrenal medulla which stimulates its receptors in many cell types throughout the body. Adrenaline is an agonist at adrenoceptors, a family of cell surface receptors whose main members (those that are important for understanding commonly used drugs) are α_1-, α_2-, β_1-, and β_2-adrenoceptors.

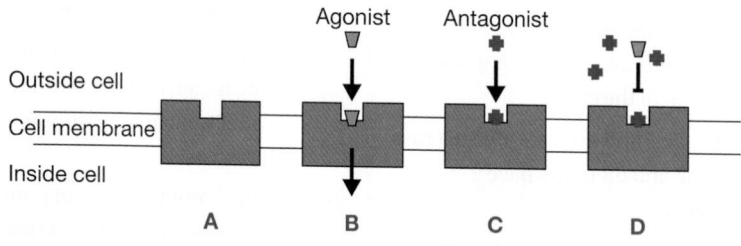

Figure 2.1 Agonist and antagonist action at a cell surface receptor.

The cell membrane is shown with the receptor in orange crossing the membrane from outside to inside the cell. In A no ligand is present (i.e. no agonist or antagonist). In B an agonist (green symbol) is present in the extracellular compartment. This could be a naturally occurring hormone or neurotransmitter, or it could be a drug. It stimulates the receptor, sending signals into the cell which change cellular function. In C an antagonist is present (blue symbol) outside the cell; it binds to the same receptor site, but does not stimulate it. Therefore the cell's function is not changed. In D the agonist is again present, but this time so are antagonist molecules. The antagonist occupies the receptor and so, despite the presence of the agonist, the receptor is not stimulated. Note that the effect of the antagonist is dependent on the presence of the agonist (compare D with C).

The following case is a clinical example of the use of a drug acting as an agonist at adrenoceptors.

> Amritpal is a pharmacy student who has asthma. She gets up early for an 8 a.m. lecture, rushes to catch the train to university, and then finds she is struggling to breathe, with wheezing and coughing. She finds her blue inhaler, takes two puffs, and within a few seconds she is breathing freely. The inhaler contains a drug called salbutamol which has a structure closely related to that of adrenaline. When Amritpal inhales the salbutamol it reaches the small airways (the bronchioles) in her lungs. During an asthmatic episode these small tubes, which have flexible walls, become too narrow. This is partly because they have smooth muscle wrapped around them that contracts, squeezing the bronchioles and making the passage of air difficult.[2] The smooth muscle cells have β_2-adrenoceptors on their surface. The salbutamol *stimulates* these receptors, i.e. it is an *agonist* at β_2-adrenoceptors. The stimulated receptors send signals inside the cell that encourage the muscle to relax, so that the airways open up and breathing becomes easier.

Now consider another case, in which an antagonist drug is used.

> Balrag is 60 years old, and has high blood pressure.[3] This means that his heart is pumping too much blood per minute against too high a resistance from the blood vessels around his body, and so the pressure in the vessels carrying blood away from the heart (the arteries) is elevated. Balrag's heart is stimulated by the hormone adrenaline, released from the adrenal medulla. His heart muscle cells have adrenoceptors on them, mainly β_1-adrenoceptors. His natural adrenaline stimulates the adrenoceptors (i.e. it is an agonist at these receptors) and this makes his heart beat more strongly, contributing to his high blood pressure. Many years ago he was prescribed a drug called atenolol, which he has taken as a tablet every morning since. It is a β_1-adrenoceptor **antagonist**. When he takes atenolol it spreads around his body, including his heart, where it competes with adrenaline to occupy the β_1-adrenoceptors. Atenolol does not stimulate these receptors, but by occupying them it prevents binding of the natural ligand adrenaline. It therefore reduces receptor stimulation mediated by adrenaline (see Figure 2.1); his heart beats less strongly, contributing to a reduced blood pressure and decreasing his risk of suffering a heart attack or stroke.

These two commonplace scenarios illustrate that both agonists and antagonists have a role to play in therapeutics.

2.1.2 The subdivision of receptors into types and subtypes is important for therapeutics

The examples above, of treatment of asthma with β_2-adrenoceptor agonists and of high blood pressure with β_1-adrenoceptor antagonists, also illustrate the importance of the study of receptor subtypes, their classification, and the development by pharmacologists and chemists of subtype-specific ligands (and potential drugs). As already stated, the major adrenoceptors in airway smooth muscle cells are β_2-adrenoceptors, while those in the heart are principally β_1-adrenoceptors. The recognition of this difference paved the way for the development of β_2-selective agonists in inhalers for asthma which were largely free of cardiac effects. In this way receptor classification revolutionized life for millions of asthma sufferers the world over, and saved countless lives (Figure 2.2).

As mentioned above, the α_1-adrenoceptors (subdivided into α_1- and α_2-adrenoceptors) are also important for clinical pharmacology, as illustrated by the following example.

> After a few years of taking his β_1-adrenoceptor antagonist, Balrag finds his blood pressure is not adequately controlled and he ends up taking several drugs. One of them is doxazosin, a selective α_1-adrenoceptor antagonist. α_1-Adrenoceptors are found on the vascular smooth muscle cells, which are wrapped around the smaller blood vessels that the heart is pumping blood through. Stimulation of these receptors by naturally occurring adrenaline (or noradrenaline) leads to constriction of the blood vessels and an increase in resistance to blood flow. This results in elevated blood pressure. When doxazosin is present it will occupy the α_1-adrenoceptors, blocking the binding of adrenaline and noradrenaline. Vasoconstriction will therefore be reduced, and so in turn will blood pressure.

Note here that by paying attention to receptor subtypes the patient is targeting his high blood pressure at two crucial locations, the pump (the heart) and the resistance to flow (small blood vessels; see also Chapter 5). With this understanding we are able to target our drugs to a particular anatomical site and a specific physiological function, and either increase the activity at the receptors (using agonists) or reduce receptor activation (using antagonists). The principal objective of treatment with any drug is to generate a highly specific effect in a particular region of the body. This can sometimes be achieved by localized administration of the drug (e.g. the use of antibiotic ointment to treat a skin infection).

---

2 This is only one of several aspects of asthma. See Chapter 11 to learn more about this condition and its treatment.

3 See Chapter 5.

10

Chapter 2 How do drugs work? An introduction

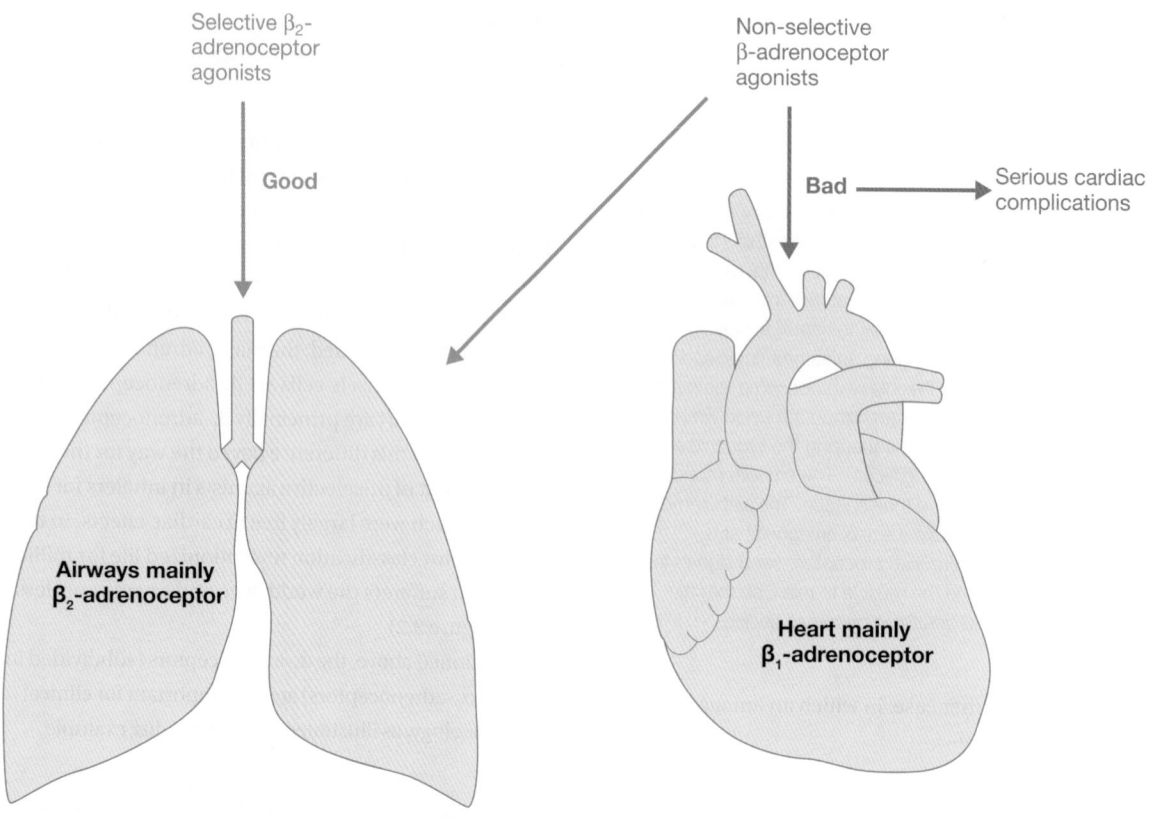

Figure 2.2 Importance of β-adrenoceptor subtypes in the treatment of asthma.

The β-adrenoceptor agonists which are selective for β_2-adrenoceptors as well as non-selective drugs acting at both β_1- and β_2-adrenoceptors will have beneficial effects in opening airways. However, the non-selective drug also has significant cardiac effects and cannot be used in the treatment of asthma. Effective and safe treatment of this respiratory disorder was enabled through an understanding of β-adrenoceptor subtypes and their differing pharmacology.

However, within the body this is generally accomplished by using drugs that are highly selective for particular receptor subtypes, as in the examples above.

2.1.3 Partial agonists show properties of both agonists and antagonists and offer flexible treatment options

Consider a strip of muscle tissue suspended from both ends in a bath of physiological fluid, so that any contraction of the muscle can be recorded and quantified. When an agonist (drug A) for a receptor present on the muscle cells is added, it stimulates contraction. Applying different concentrations of the agonist will give different sized responses. This will generate data which can be plotted as a concentration–response curve, i.e. the relationship between the concentration of drug A present, and the response it elicits. A typical curve is shown in Figure 2.3 for drug A (blue line).

It can be seen that the response becomes larger as more agonist is added, but only up to a certain point—beyond this the response remains the same despite the addition of more drug. A plateau is reached. This is because drug A can only generate a response when it is bound to the receptor—in effect when it **occupies** the receptor. When there is no drug present, none of the receptors are occupied and the response size is zero. As the concentration of drug A around the receptors increases, more of the drug binds to the receptors and the size of the response increases. However, there must be a fixed number of receptors on this piece of tissue, so as we continue to increase the concentration of drug A eventually it will occupy all of the available receptors. Increasing the concentration of drug A further will not increase the size of the response, since all the receptors are now occupied and fully stimulated; a plateau is formed at the top of the concentration–response curve.

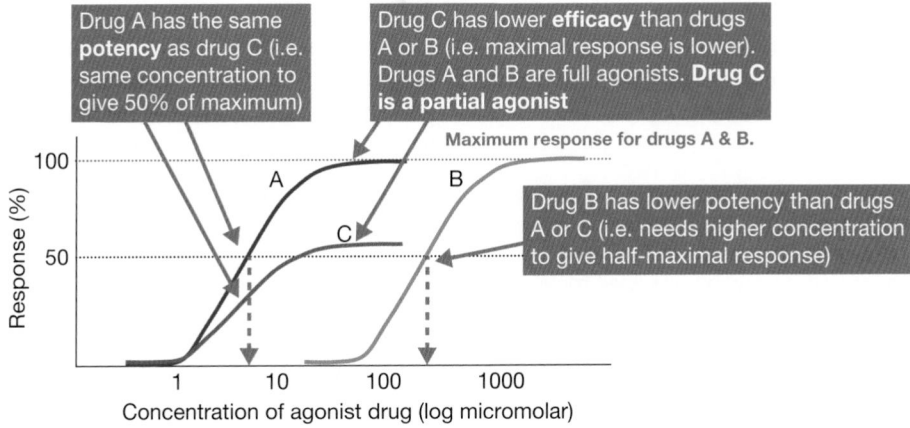

Figure 2.3 Concentration–response curves for three different agonists, all of which act on the same population of receptors to generate the response.

Drugs A and B are both full agonists. Drug A is more potent than drug B. Drug C is a partial agonist. It has the same EC_{50} as drug A, so it has equal potency, but it can only give a fraction of the maximal response that drug A can give, i.e. drug C has a lower efficacy than drug A.

The binding/occupation issues are explored further later in this chapter (Figures 2.5 and 2.6).

Returning to our experimental situation, Figure 2.3 shows concentration–response curves for two additional drugs (B and C) added to the fluid immersing the strip of muscle. Note that all three drugs act on the same receptor population. If we add drug B instead of drug A, the same maximum contractile response is generated but this requires a higher concentration of drug. It is helpful to consider the concentration of drug which gives **half the maximal response** (the EC_{50}). Compared with drug A, drug B requires a higher concentration to give half the maximal response, so the EC_{50} for drug B is *higher* than the EC_{50} for drug A. We say that drug A has a higher **potency** than drug B because we can achieve 50% of the maximal response with a *lower* concentration.

Now look at the concentration–response curve for drug C in Figure 2.3. It also reaches a plateau, but this is lower than that for drug A. However much drug C we add we can never get as big a response as we can with drug A. And yet these two drugs have the same EC_{50}. (Note that the EC_{50} is the concentration giving half the maximal response for *that* drug.) We make two observations.

1) The lower plateau for drug C is evidence that drug C has a lower **efficacy** than drug A. When it occupies the receptor it does not stimulate it as strongly.

2) The two drugs have the same potency. We know this because the concentration required to give half the maximal response (the EC_{50}) is the same.

So drug C can give a response. It binds to the same receptors as drug A and acts as an agonist, but it cannot give a full response. It is a **partial agonist**, in contrast with drugs A and B, which are called **full agonists**.

This may be useful in itself. You may want a drug which has an effect, but which is not as powerful as some other drugs.

Steve is a patient with moderate but quite troubling persistent abdominal pain. His condition is stable, and he is at home, but he finds that ibuprofen does not adequately control his pain. His doctor wants to give him an opiate (i.e. morphine-like) drug, but knows that moderate pain does not warrant such a powerful drug with such addiction/abuse potential. A number of options are available;[4] one he considers is a drug called buprenorphine. This acts at the same receptors as morphine, but it is a partial agonist. Relating this example to Figure 2.3, morphine is drug A and buprenorphine is drug C, and the response is pain reduction. Buprenorphine gives less maximal pain relief but is sufficient for the moderate pain experienced by Steve, and he becomes more comfortable.

4 See Chapter 20, where the management of pain with drugs is explored.

Here a partial agonist was more appropriate than a full agonist. A partial agonist has another feature which is illustrated by our experimental example, where both drug A and drug C are binding at the same receptor site.

> Joe is a drug addict. He regularly takes heroin, a drug closely related to morphine and which acts on the same receptors. He has a sufficient supply of heroin to take frequently, so as to prevent the horrible effects of withdrawal (see Chapter 20). Sometimes he takes other drugs as well. On this day he takes a new drug stolen from a clinic. He doesn't know it, but has taken buprenorphine. He immediately starts to become very ill—he is rapidly precipitated into partial withdrawal.

Buprenorphine binds very strongly to the same receptor as heroin; if heroin is also present, buprenorphine will displace it from the receptor. But as it is only a partial agonist it will produce a much lower level of response from the receptors than the heroin that it displaces, precipitating withdrawal. Buprenorphine is acting as an **antagonist** in the presence of heroin.

A partial agonist, then, can also act as an antagonist when given at the same time as a full agonist, binding to the receptor and reducing the response to the full agonist, as illustrated by this example and diagrammatically in Figure 2.4. From this figure we can see that drug C exhibits both agonist and antagonist behaviour, but because it has some agonist activity it is not a **pure antagonist**.

2.1.4 What determines the potency of drugs: efficacy and affinity

We have already considered the term 'potency' when looking at the response curves to agonists in Figure 2.3. It is this which determines the concentration of an agonist drug that is needed to produce a given size of response. A drug's potency, therefore, has a major influence on its clinical effect, and so it is obviously important that we have some understanding of what determines it.

As we have already said, the drugs we are considering are ligands that bind to receptors and stimulate them to different degrees. Pure antagonists do not stimulate the receptors at all, whereas maximally effective concentrations of full agonists stimulate them to produce the largest response possible. We use the term **efficacy**[5] to describe this attribute—the ability of a drug, once bound to the receptor, to stimulate it and bring about a response. Further aspects of efficacy and what it tells us about how drugs and receptors work are considered in Box 2.2.

A separate but equally important property of drugs is how *tightly* they bind to their receptors—some drugs bind more strongly than others. A drug that binds very strongly to its receptor is said to have a high **affinity**. In our example above, the partial agonist buprenorphine binds *very* strongly to the opiate (morphine) receptor (see Chapter 20, Section 20.3.1) and yet cannot fully activate it. Many pure antagonists have a high affinity for receptors binding very strongly but, as antagonists, causing no activation. These examples illustrate the point that binding and activation are two different things, which we need to comprehend to understand how drugs work. We introduced the binding/occupation of drugs and

---

5 Strictly speaking we should use the term 'intrinsic efficacy' to describe the attribute of the drug which results in the size of the response at the level of the receptor, but here we will be satisfied with a simplified terminology. It is also worth noting that in a clinical setting the term 'efficacy' may be used in a much broader sense than here, i.e. to describe how effective a drug is at generating a desirable clinical outcome.

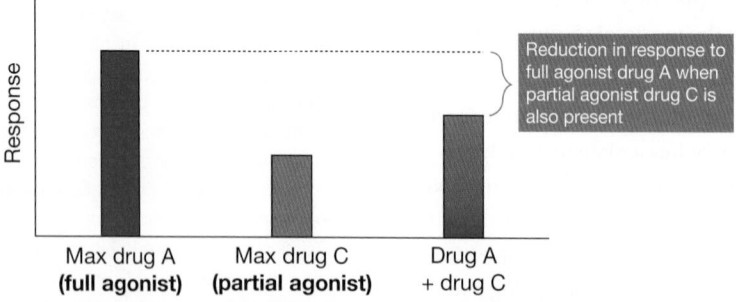

Figure 2.4 Drug A is a full agonist and drug C is a partial agonist at the same population of receptors.

Both are used at their maximally effective concentration (see Figure 2.3). When the two drugs are added together some of the receptors will be occupied by drug A and some by drug C. The final response will be lower than that produced by drug A alone, meaning that drug C appears to be working like an antagonist.

Box 2.2

Receptor reserve, efficacy, and irreversible antagonists

For an agonist to give a response at a receptor it must occupy it. As explained in the text (Section 2.1.4) an equilibrium is established, with free agonist (i.e. in solution) constantly exchanging with bound molecules (i.e. attached to cell surface receptors).

We also know that occupation of receptors alone is not enough to give a response—an antagonist can occupy exactly the same binding site but give no response. The additional factor, what the agonist *does* to the receptor to turn it on, is called efficacy (see this chapter, footnote 5).

We can gain an interesting insight into how agonist drugs work by comparing the binding of a drug, its occupation curve, to its concentration–response curve, as in Figure b. The striking thing is that the response curve is not the same as the occupancy curve—it lies to the left.

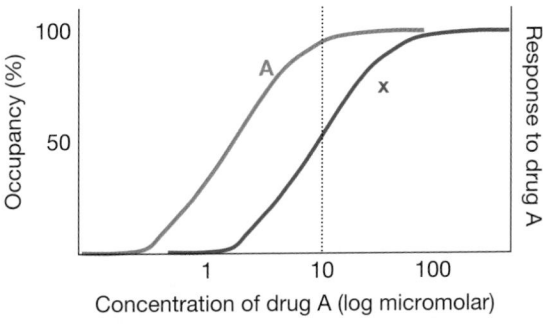

Figure b The occupation curve and the concentration–response curve for an agonist are often not the same.

The blue line (X) is the occupation curve for agonist drug A, and the red line (A) is its concentration–response curve. The dotted line shows that only 50% of receptors are occupied at a concentration of 10 μM, yet this is able to produce a maximal response.

Examining Figure b closely, we can see that we get a full response with only 50% occupancy of the receptors. This occurs at a drug concentration of 10 micromolar (μM). As we increase the concentration beyond this, more receptors are occupied but there is no increase in the size of the response. This may seem odd: if we are occupying more receptors, why does the response not get larger? Pharmacologists describe this as a 'receptor reserve', or they may say that there are 'spare receptors'. This is simply a way of saying that there are more receptors than needed to give a full response—stimulating half the receptors at any moment in time is sufficient to give a full response.

So what would happen if we were to reduce the number of receptors to remove the surplus? If this were done precisely, then it would mean that all receptors would need to be occupied to give a full response; the occupancy and response curves would be the same. By using an irreversible competitive antagonist receptors can effectively be removed from the available pool. This type of molecule binds to the same site as the agonist but does not dissociate from it, so that receptors cannot subsequently be activated. (Remember, most clinically used drugs are **reversible**, not irreversible competitive antagonists.) What would happen then if we took the situation in Figure b and added increasing concentrations of an irreversible antagonist? The result is shown in Figure c. As the concentration of irreversible antagonist is increased, the number of receptors available is decreased. The concentration–response curve shifts to the right as the receptor reserve is depleted. Eventually the response curve becomes identical with the occupation curve—to get a full response all receptors must now be stimulated. If we carry on increasing the

concentration of the antagonist beyond this point there will not be enough receptors, even when all are stimulated, to generate a full response; the maximum of the curve will be reduced and the curve will collapse, as shown in Figure c.

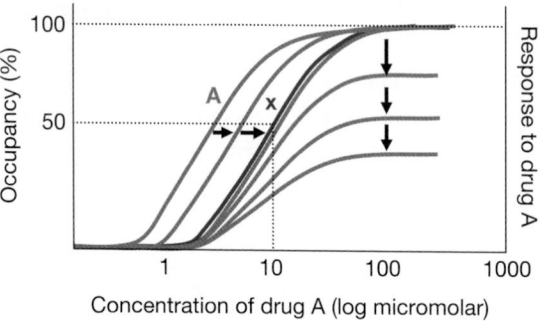

Figure c Effect of an irreversible competitive antagonist.

The blue line (X) is the occupation curve for drug A, and the far left red line (A) is its concentration–response curve. The additional red lines show the effect on the concentration–response curve of increasing concentrations (indicated by the arrows) of an irreversible competitive antagonist.

Let us examine the significance of the efficacy of our agonist a little further by returning to the situation depicted in Figure b. Consider a second agonist, B, which has the same *affinity* for the receptors and therefore the same occupation curve as drug A, but has a greater *efficacy*. This situation is shown in Figure d.

The drug with the higher efficacy does not give a bigger maximum response than the lower efficacy drug A, since both are full agonists, but it does generate this response at a lower concentration. This type of observation is of obvious clinical importance—drug B is more *potent* than drug A.

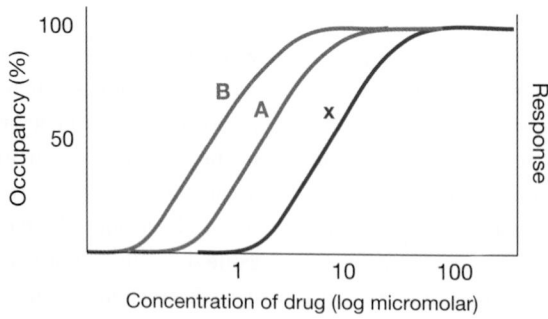

Figure d Comparison of drug A with a higher efficacy drug, B.

It is assumed that the two drugs have the same affinity for the receptor, and therefore the occupation curve in blue (X) is the same for both drugs. However, the efficacy of drug B is greater than that of drug A, and the maximal effect is achieved at a lower concentration.

receptors above (Section 2.1.3), and these ideas are now developed further. This is important when we consider how drugs work in the clinic, since clinical outcome so often deals with the competition for receptors between introduced drugs and native ligands.

The affinity of a drug for its receptor: binding is an equilibrium business

Pharmacologists have devised ways of measuring the binding of drugs to receptors. Given that receptors are specific cellular proteins, there are a limited number of binding sites on any one cell, or in any given tissue. Therefore if we expose our cells to increasing concentrations of drug (the ligand), more will bind until we have saturated the receptors (i.e. they are all occupied).

There is a danger that this gives the impression that a ligand binds to and sticks to a receptor, making it unavailable for future binding. This is not the case, at least not for natural ligands (e.g. neurotransmitters and

hormones), nor indeed for the vast majority of drugs. When one of these ligands is present in the solution bathing the receptor it binds **reversibly**, so that individual molecules of the ligand first bind to and then free themselves (dissociate) from the receptor. They are then available to bind again. This 'on–off' binding has well-understood **kinetics**: the rate at which the molecule binds to and the rate at which it dissociates from the receptor. There is an **equilibrium** between bound and free ligands (illustrated in Figure 2.5).

The balance of this equilibrium will differ depending on the properties of the ligands involved. Some will have kinetics that shift the equilibrium in favour of their binding, but it is still an on–off process so that the receptor is available for different ligands to bind to it. Pharmacologists measure these processes, coming up with an index of how strongly ligands bind. In Figure 2.6 the blue line indicates the amount of binding of drug A to the receptors as the concentration of the drug increases until it reaches a maximum, denoted as 100% binding

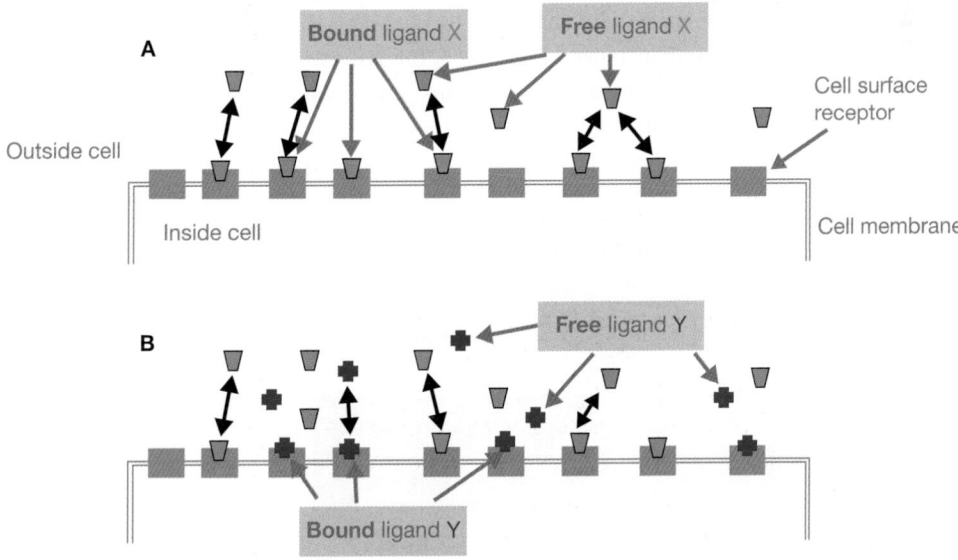

Figure 2.5 Free and bound ligands are in equilibrium and compete with each other.

Free ligand is in solution in the extracellular space. **Bound ligand** is temporarily attached to the receptors at the cell membrane. Bound molecules interchange with free molecules, going on and off the receptors repeatedly—there is an **equilibrium** between the two. There are only a limited number of receptors. In **panel A** the cell is exposed only to ligand (drug) X, shown by the **green** symbols. There are both bound and free ligands, and not all receptors are occupied. In **panel B** the cell is exposed to two ligands (drugs), X and Y, which can both occupy the same receptors. The **blue** symbols represent ligand Y. When Y is added together with X, it **competes** with X for occupation of receptors. The result is that a mixture of both X and Y occupies the receptors. Therefore Y acts to displace some of X from binding, so that overall less X is bound. The action of drug Y is **competitive**: if the affinity of Y for the receptor was greater, there would be even less binding of X. Note that if X is an agonist, and Y is a pure antagonist, there will be less **response** to X when Y is added, and even less response if Y has a greater affinity than X.

16

Chapter 2 How do drugs work? An introduction

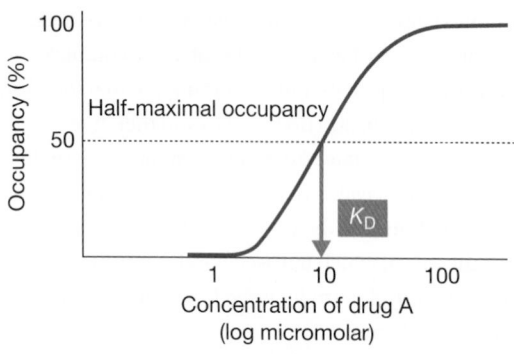

Figure 2.6 Occupancy of the receptor by a ligand is concentration dependent.

The concentration which gives half the maximum is a measure of how strongly the ligand binds to the receptor, and is designated the dissociation constant K_D. The K_D in the example here is 10 µM (10^{-5} M).

(meaning that all the receptors are now occupied by the drug).

The position of the binding curve along the concentration axis (Figure 2.6) is an indication of the strength of binding. This can be represented numerically, for comparative purposes, as the concentration giving 50% of the maximum binding (or 50% saturation). So a drug with an on–off equilibrium that gives strong binding will generate 50% saturation at a lower concentration than one that is only weakly bound. This is a measure of affinity, and is expressed as the dissociation constant K_D, as illustrated in Figure 2.6. A drug with a high affinity will reach 50% occupancy at a low concentration, and so will have a low K_D value.

Returning to Figure 2.5, we see that if there is more than one ligand in the vicinity of the receptor they will compete with each other in trying to bind to the receptor. A ligand with a low K_D, and therefore high affinity, will bind more effectively than a ligand with a low affinity (high K_D). So, for a drug to have a major effect at a low dose it needs to have a high affinity for its target receptor. It is no wonder that pharmaceutical companies attach considerable importance to the K_D of drugs under development, since most of them act at receptors in competition with the natural ligand (e.g. neurotransmitter or hormone).

Note that the consideration of affinity relates to drugs that are agonists and antagonists, whereas efficacy issues only apply to drugs that are agonists (because a pure antagonist has, by definition, no efficacy).

2.1.5 Back to antagonists: reversible and irreversible competition

We have said that antagonists reduce the effect of an agonist by **competing reversibly** for the same binding sites. This idea is illustrated in both Figure 2.1 and Figure 2.5. This is the way most clinically useful antagonists work; such drugs are called **reversible competitive antagonists**. To explore this further, consider a concentration–response curve for an agonist. What happens to this curve if we add a reversible competitive antagonist to the agonist?

The notable thing about Figure 2.7 is that the concentration–response curve for agonist A reaches the same maximum in the presence of the antagonist, but the curve is shifted to the

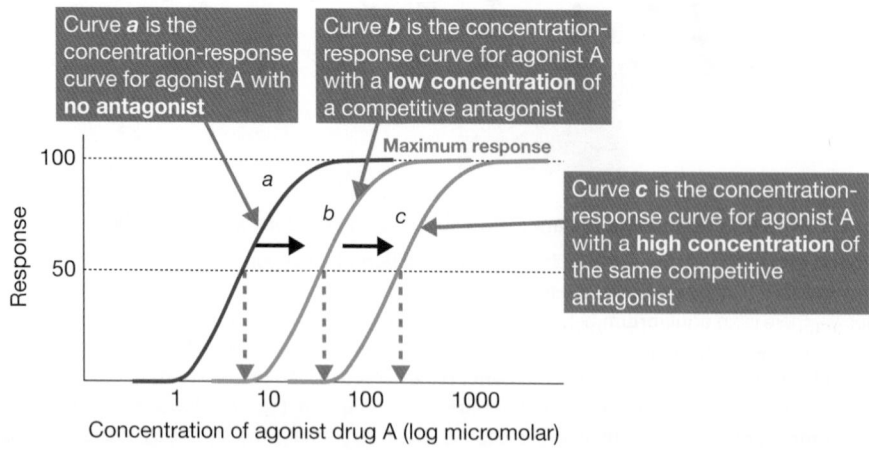

Figure 2.7 Three concentration–response curves for a single agonist A in the absence of an antagonist (curve a), and in the presence of a reversible competitive antagonist at low concentration (curve b) or high concentration (curve c).

right; the concentration of A required to reach the maximum is higher in the presence of the competitor drug. What this means is that a reversible competitive antagonist will not reduce the response to a natural agonist that is at a very high concentration.

> Clare suffers from hay fever. When the pollen count rises she takes antihistamines. She finds that many of her symptoms are reduced if she takes the antihistamines early enough, but the distressing itchiness and swelling of the tissue around her eyes do not seem to be helped by the drug.

The antihistamines used to treat hay fever are competitive antagonists. Hay fever is caused in part by histamine released from cells called mast cells, which are concentrated in parts of the body exposed to the environment, like the skin, particularly that around the eyes. Mast cells release a large amount of histamine when stimulated by pollen, for example, and it is likely that part of the reason Clare does not get relief from these symptoms is that the histamine concentration at its receptors is so high that it out-competes the antihistamine drug. The drug can't bind, so it has no effect.

Since most clinical drugs are competitive antagonists, the ideas introduced here have a widespread influence on the effectiveness of drug-based therapies.

Irreversible competitive antagonists bind to the same site on the receptor as the agonist but, unlike reversible antagonists, they do not then dissociate from the receptor, which therefore cannot be activated. This type of antagonism, though, has few clinical applications. As such, the term 'competitive antagonist' is often used to describe drugs which bind reversibly.

Non-competitive antagonists reduce receptor stimulation by binding elsewhere on the receptor molecule and not to the agonist binding site. As such, they do not compete with the agonist for binding, hence the term non-competitive. This type of antagonist could, for instance, prevent conformational changes in the receptor which are required for its activation following agonist binding. Like irreversible competitive antagonists they have a more profound effect on the maximal response which, under many circumstances, will be lower, even at the highest concentration of agonist. Non-competitive antagonism is not very common amongst therapeutic agents.

2.2 How receptor activation changes cells

Drugs that act at receptors either activate them (agonists such as salbutamol used in asthma) or prevent their activation (antagonists such as atenolol used in high blood pressure); if we want to understand therapeutics we need to know how the receptors work.

The receptor, when activated by a native agonist, such as a neurotransmitter or a hormone, or by an agonist drug, must send a signal into the cell that changes the function of the cell in some way. There are a very large number of ways in which receptors do this. Here, we introduce a few that are encountered in the clinical context of the rest of this book.

Receptors are located either on the surface of cells or inside the cells. Firstly, we will provide an overview of some of the many mechanisms activated by **cell surface** receptors.

2.2.1 Cell surface receptors: some examples with different effector mechanisms

There are a huge number of cell surface receptors with widely different structures. One thing they all have in common is that they are intrinsic proteins of the cell membrane, which means that they cross the cell membrane and therefore have an extracellular domain, a transmembrane domain, and an intracellular domain. Figure 2.8 illustrates some of the common structures of the cell surface receptor proteins.

Pharmacologists classify receptors in a number of different, overlapping, and not necessarily logically organized ways. Features which guide classification include the native agonist(s), the mechanism by which they operate, the relative affinity of other ligands, including antagonists, and structural relationships revealed by molecular biology. For example, acetylcholine receptors (AChRs) include ligand-gated ion channels and G protein-coupled receptors (GPCRs). These two classes of AChR are, for historical reasons, named after the plant/fungus-derived agonist drugs nicotine (from the tobacco plant) and muscarine (found in one species of poisonous mushroom); the ligand-gated ion channel is therefore called the **nicotinic acetylcholine receptor** (**nAChR**) and the GPCR is termed the **muscarinic acetylcholine receptor** (**mAChR**).

18

Chapter 2 How do drugs work? An introduction

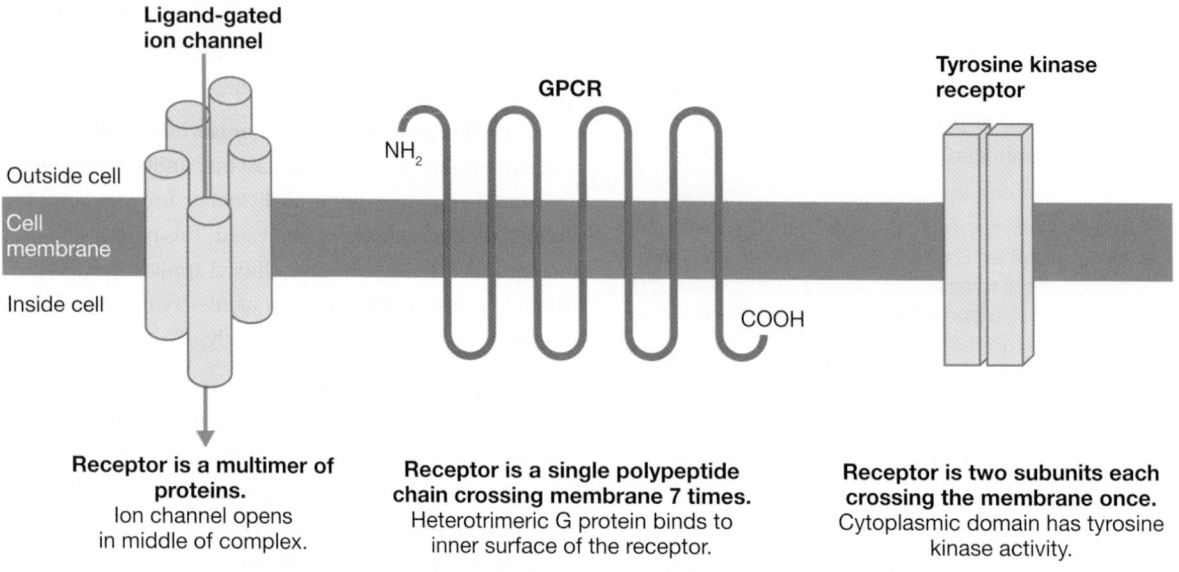

Figure 2.8 Three different types of cell surface receptor.

In each case the cartoon of the protein crossing the membrane (in orange) shows the presence of an extracellular domain poking out of the membrane into the extracellular space, a transmembrane domain, which may involve multiple crossings of the membrane by one or more polypeptide chains, and an intracellular domain. GPCR, G protein-coupled receptor.

Ligand-gated ion channels and GPCRs account for most of the cell surface receptors we encounter in clinical pharmacology. We will also consider here the mechanism of action of the insulin receptor, which operates in a manner used by classical growth factor receptors, collectively called tyrosine kinase receptors. In limiting the account in this section to these three mechanisms—ligand-gated, GPCR, and tyrosine kinase receptors (Figure 2.8)—we must not forget that there are many other important mechanisms whereby cell surface receptors regulate cellular function.

2.2.2 Ligand-gated ion channel receptors

Ligand-gated ion channels are commonly found in excitable cells, essentially meaning muscle and nerve cells. One of their important characteristics is the fast speed at which they can deliver signals, and this underlies their localization to areas where rapid response (e.g. skeletal muscle) or fast information processing (e.g. the brain) is required. All cells have gradients of ions across the cell membrane at rest, and for excitable cells this means they are often capable of firing action potentials, during which rapid changes in these gradients occur. The ligand-gated ion channel receptor is composed of several

subunits that cross the membrane, clustered together to form a pore or ion channel in the middle (Figure 2.8). On binding of the agonist to the extracellular domain of the receptor complex, a conformational change occurs and the subunits pull apart to open the ion channel. (This transition between the open and closed state of the ion channel is termed **gating**; for ligand-gated channels it is brought about by the agonist binding, whereas voltage-gated channels open and close in response to changes in potential across the plasma membrane.)

The channels also have **selectivity**, which means that they are selective for the ions they let through which include Na^+, Ca^{2+}, K^+, or Cl^- ions. When the channels are open, ions move according to the concentration gradient, from where it is higher on one side of the membrane to the other. For example, Na^+ is normally lower inside the cell (the cytosol) than outside, so opening a Na^+ channel will let the ion flow into the cell. Figure 2.9 illustrates this for a ligand-gated channel selective for Na^+; when the ligand binds, the channel opens and Na^+ flows in. Where there is a voltage difference across the membrane this will also affect the flow of ions, for example with positively charged ions attracted to the negatively charged side of the membrane.

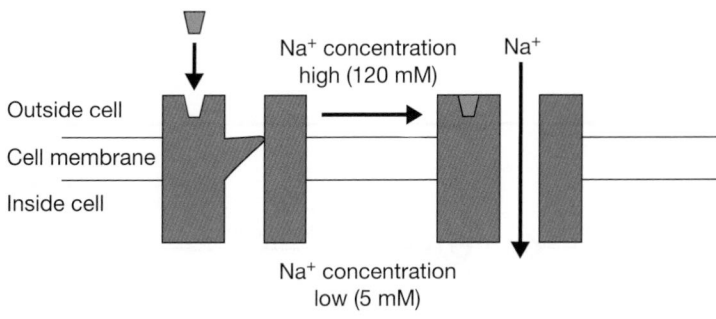

Figure 2.9 Ligand-gated ion channels.

The ion channel has a binding site for the agonist (green symbol). When this site is empty (left) the ion channel is closed, but when it is occupied by the agonist (right) the channel flips open. Channels have selectivity, in this case for Na^+, and this determines the consequences of opening the ion channel. In the example shown, the channel is selective for Na^+, which is higher outside the cell than inside, and therefore agonist binding allows Na^+ into the cell, making the inside of the membrane more positive, i.e. the membrane depolarizes.

We shall consider the nicotinic acetylcholine receptor (nAChR) as an example of a ligand-gated ion channel.

nAChR is a ligand-gated channel for Na^+, as shown in Figure 2.9. This means that acetylcholine (ACh) acting at this receptor in a nerve or muscle cell will always be excitatory. This is because an excitable cell will always have more Na^+ outside the cell than inside, so when the nAChR is operated, the inside of the cell will become less negative, stimulating the nerve cell to form action potentials, or leading to the muscle contracting. It is the nAChR at the neuromuscular junction that is stimulated by ACh released by motor neurons to mediate all skeletal muscle contraction.

The autonomic nervous system controls nearly all aspects of bodily function apart from skeletal muscle, and is composed of sympathetic and parasympathetic branches. In both branches messages are carried from the central nervous system (CNS) via two neurons which form a synapse at the ganglia. ACh is released from the terminals of the pre-ganglionic neuron to stimulate nAChR on the cell body of the post-ganglionic neuron; this is the case in both the sympathetic and parasympathetic nervous systems. The action potential generated as a consequence of the influx of Na^+ carries the signal on towards the effector cells/tissue. At the final synapse between the post-ganglionic neuron terminals and the effector cells, there are differences between the branches of the autonomic nervous systems, as shown in Figure 2.10. In the case of the parasympathetic nervous system, ACh is again released from the post-ganglionic neuron, but here acts on *muscarinic* acetylcholine receptors (mAChR) on the target cells. In contrast, almost all post-ganglionic neurons in the sympathetic nervous system release noradrenaline, which then acts on adrenoceptors on the target tissue. There are many subtypes of adrenoceptor and mAChR, but all are G protein-coupled receptors (see below); any given cell expresses a specific complement of these which determines the response to messages relayed from the CNS via the two branches of the autonomic nervous system.

Brain ligand-gated ion channel receptors: glutamate and GABA, accelerators and brakes

There are also some nAChRs in the brain. Their role is poorly defined and they have no direct impact on our understanding of therapeutics, so they are not considered further here. However, the brain does depend on glutamate receptors, which are also ligand-gated ion channels. These glutamate receptors, illustrated in Chapter 16 (Box 16.1, Figure b), are excitatory (the channel selectivity is for Na^+ and Ca^{2+}), and it is this excitatory neurotransmission that underlies brain activity—without it our brains would not work. Some of the fascinating complexities of brain glutamate and gamma-aminobutyric acid (GABA) ion channel receptors, and the possibilities for drug interaction, are introduced in later chapters in Part 5. The central importance in the brain of ligand-gated ion channels is

20

Chapter 2 How do drugs work? An introduction

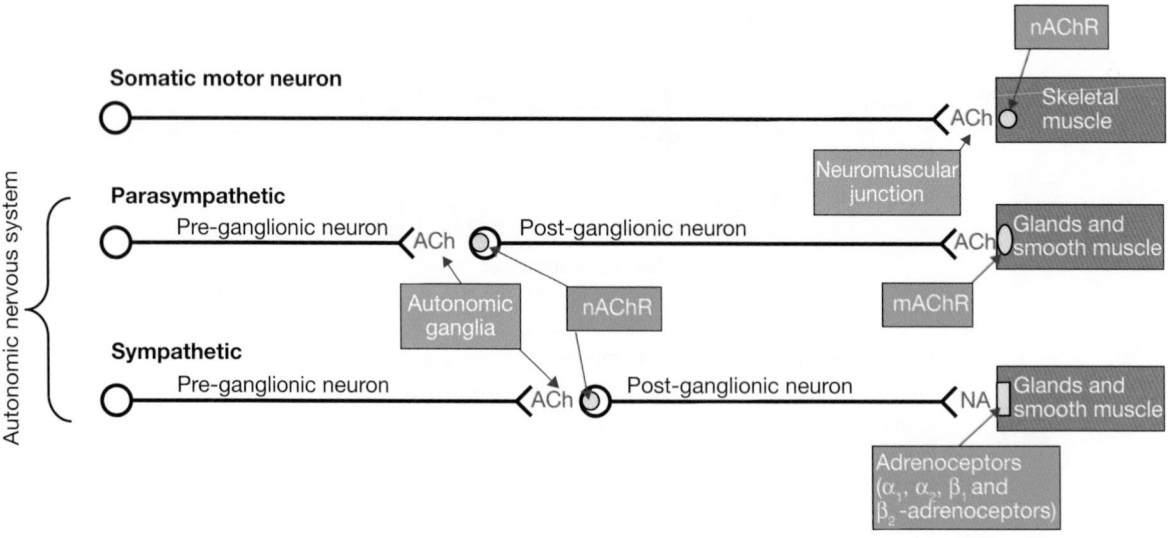

Figure 2.10 The location of receptors for acetylcholine and noradrenaline (norepinephrine) in the somatic nervous system, and the sympathetic and parasympathetic branches of the autonomic nervous system.

Note that in the somatic nervous system, a single motor neuron directly innervates skeletal muscle. ACh is released from its terminals at the neuromuscular junction, and acts on nAChRs on the skeletal muscle fibres to cause contraction. In both branches of the autonomic nervous system, ACh is released from the pre-ganglionic neurons and acts on nAChRs located on the cell bodies of the post-ganglionic neurons. In the parasympathetic nervous system, these post-ganglionic cells again release ACh, but here it acts on muscarinic ACh receptors on the target cells (red boxes). In contrast, almost all post-ganglionic neurons in the sympathetic nervous system release noradrenaline, which acts on adrenoceptors expressed by the target cells. ACh, acetylcholine; nAChR, nicotinic acetylcholine receptor; mAChR, muscarinic acetylcholine receptor; NA, noradrenaline (norepinephrine).

not limited to glutamate receptors. If these are the accelerator pedal of the brain, then we need a brake pedal as well, and this is provided by the neurotransmitter GABA, acting on the ligand-gated ion channel $GABA_A$ receptors (see Chapter 16, Box 16.1, for more on accelerators and brakes in the brain). They are selective for K^+ ions, and since these are at a higher concentration inside the cell than outside, GABA-induced opening of the channel allows K^+ to flow out of the cell. As the positive charge moves across the membrane the neuron's resting potential (negative on the inside) is kept low, and action potential generation is less likely.

2.2.3 G protein-coupled receptors

GPCRs are a superfamily of receptors that have two principal characteristics.

1) They consist of a single polypeptide chain which crosses the cell membrane seven times (they are sometimes referred to as seven-transmembrane (7TM) receptors), with an extracellular N-terminus and an intracellular C-terminal tail (Figure 2.8).

2) They send signals into the cell through an agonist-controlled interaction with a G protein at the inner face of the cell membrane. The G protein specifically interacts with the third intracellular loop of the receptor.

Heterotrimeric G proteins

G proteins act as the interface between receptor activation by an agonist, and the response generated inside the cell which is being stimulated. Each G protein comprises three different subunits, denoted α, β, and γ (hence 'heterotrimeric'). The G protein recognizes activated receptors and acts to pass on the signal to the enzymes and/or ion channels (effectors) that are the ultimate targets of GPCRs. It is usually the activation or inhibition of these target proteins which gives rise to the response to stimulation of GPCRs (Figure 2.11).

Heterotrimeric G proteins are not all the same: different G proteins link to different receptors and interact with specific effectors. These associations are, though, specific to the particular GPCR involved and the cell type

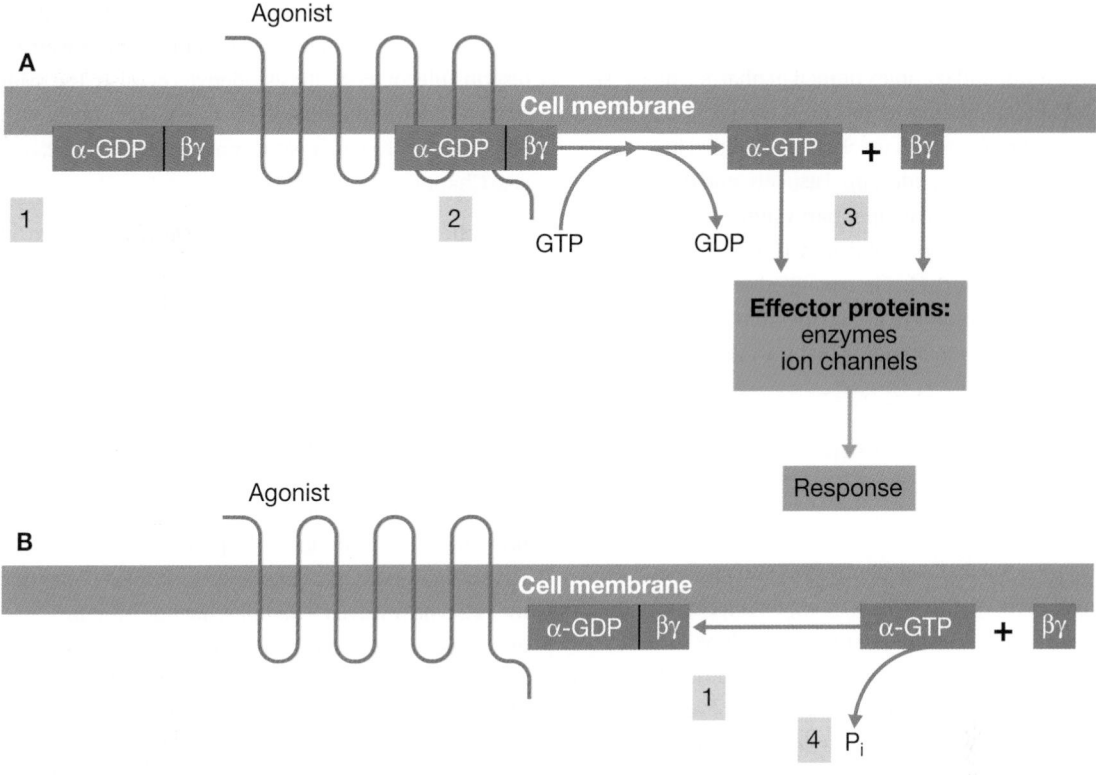

Figure 2.11 Heterotrimeric G protein function.

Panel A The blue symbols represent the G protein, initially in its resting state as a heterotrimer of α-GDP, β, and γ subunits all associated with each other [1]. Following its activation by the agonist, a conformational change in the receptor increases its affinity for the G protein, which moves in the lipid bilayer to interact with the receptor at the G protein binding region (third intracellular loop) [2]. This interaction leads to the α subunit losing its affinity for GDP and gaining affinity for GTP. The GTP-bound α subunit dissociates from the βγ subunits which remain associated with each other. Both α-GTP and βγ then interact with the enzymes and ion channels to bring about the response of the cell to the agonist [3]. **Panel B** The signal is turned off through the built-in GTPase activity of the α subunit which converts the bound GTP to GDP [4]. With GDP bound, the α subunit again associates with the βγ subunits, and the G protein is then available once more for activation by the agonist–receptor complex [1].

that it is expressed in. In this way different GPCRs are coupled selectively to different responses.

A G protein has a single pocket that can be filled with either guanosine-5′-diphosphate (GDP) or guanosine-5′-triphosphate (GTP). (It is this interaction with guanosine nucleotides that accounts for the term G protein.) The G protein is activated when the pocket is filled with the small molecule GTP, but is inactive when GDP is attached. In a heterotrimeric G protein the GDP/GTP pocket is in the α subunit. When an agonist binds to a GPCR, there is a change in conformation of the receptor which favours its interaction with the G protein. This in turn leads to the dissociation of the GDP molecule from the α subunit, which is replaced by GTP. With the GTP attached, the α subunit separates from

the βγ subunits (which remain associated). Both the α-GTP subunit and the βγ subunits may then regulate enzymes or ion channels (Figure 2.11). In this way, G proteins act as intermediaries between the activated receptors and the effector proteins which ultimately change the way the cell behaves. Amplification is built into the system as an activated receptor interacts repeatedly with many G proteins, and these interact with effectors for long enough to generate many molecules of product.

The signal is terminated by the built-in GTPase activity of the α subunit, which rapidly hydrolyses GTP to GDP. This allows the reassociation of α and βγ subunits, and the complex is then available to enter the cycle again (Figure 2.11, Panel B).

22

Chapter 2 How do drugs work? An introduction

This account of the way in which GPCRs change cell function is a highly simplified account of what has become a vast and complex branch of pharmacology (see recommended reading, at the end of each chapter). The heterotrimeric G protein mechanism outlined in Figure 2.11 has many additional aspects, and the issue of GPCRs operating in a manner partly independent of G proteins has also been established. However, the central story told in Figure 2.11, when coupled with a discussion of the effector proteins (e.g. enzymes and ion channels), is sufficient for understanding many aspects of drug use in the clinic.

2.2.4 Second messengers, protein phosphorylation, and cellular regulation by GPCRs

One of the ways that activation of cell surface receptors changes events within cells is by regulating enzymes that generate molecules, referred to collectively as **second messengers**. These then act within the same cell to control different aspects of cell function. They are often water soluble and diffuse a short distance within the cytosol to reach target proteins, but some are lipid based and stay within the membrane. Agonists (first messengers) therefore stimulate receptors at the cell surface, leading to the formation of second messengers, which act as signalling molecules to carry the signal into the cell and bring about changes as directed by the agonist.

Commonly, the second messengers themselves activate **protein kinases**, enzymes which phosphorylate proteins. In so doing they change protein function, altering the way in which the cell or tissue behaves to bring about the physiological response, such as muscle contraction or gland secretion.

Here we shall introduce two GPCR-regulated enzyme systems that control most cells in the body, and which we will frequently encounter in the clinical material that follows. These are (1) the systems which regulate **cyclic AMP** synthesis, and (2) activation of **phospholipase C**.

GPCR control of cyclic AMP synthesis underlies much drug action. Let us consider our asthma patient Amritpal, whom we encountered earlier. When she inhaled salbutamol her asthma symptoms were quickly relieved. We mentioned above that salbutamol acts as an agonist at the β_2-adrenoceptors on the surface of the smooth muscle cells which wrap around the small airways. Stimulation of these receptors sends signals into the cell, causing the muscle to relax. The major signalling molecule involved here is cyclic AMP; stimulation of the β_2-adrenoceptors increases its intracellular level by stimulating the enzyme responsible for its synthesis, adenylyl cyclase. The result is the relaxation of the smooth muscle in the bronchioles, enabling Amritpal to breathe more easily (Figure 2.12; see also Chapter 11).

A number of types of heterotrimeric G proteins have been identified. The β_2-adrenoceptors are coupled to cyclic AMP synthesis by G_s, and it is the freed α_s-GTP subunit that leads to increased cyclic AMP synthesis. Once its levels in the cytosol are raised, cyclic AMP stimulates protein kinase A which phosphorylates target proteins. This coupling of activated receptors to increased intracellular cyclic AMP levels through G_s is extremely common, and occurs in most cells. Once activated, protein kinase A stimulates the phosphorylation of a large variety of proteins, the exact nature of which depends on the cell type involved. Examples include proteins associated with muscle contractile mechanisms, and ion channels (e.g. those controlling entry of Ca^{2+} into cells). The result of increases in cyclic AMP levels in the case of bronchiolar smooth muscle cells is relaxation (see Figure 2.12). However, it should be noted that the response in other muscle cells may be the opposite, as when contractility is increased in heart muscle cells (myocytes) following stimulation of G_s-coupled β_1-receptors.

In this account agonists stimulate receptors which *raise* cyclic AMP synthesis. It should be noted, however, that adenylyl cyclase is always active inside cells; its rate of activity can therefore be both increased and decreased. Indeed, there are a very large number of receptors that are coupled through a different G protein, G_i, which results its *inhibition*; activation of these receptors leads to a *reduction* in cyclic AMP levels (Figure 2.13).

Of particular note here is that both the increase and the decrease in cyclic AMP synthesis are due to **agonists** acting on their respective receptors—whether it goes up or down depends on the G protein (G_s or G_i) to which that receptor couples. The agonist can be either the natural ligand for the receptor, such as a neurotransmitter or hormone, or a therapeutic drug.

Drugs may also increase cyclic AMP levels by reducing its breakdown: phosphodiesterase inhibitors

Cyclic AMP is destroyed in the cytosol by enzymes called phosphodiesterases. When considering drugs it is possible, therefore, to raise cyclic AMP levels not only by increasing

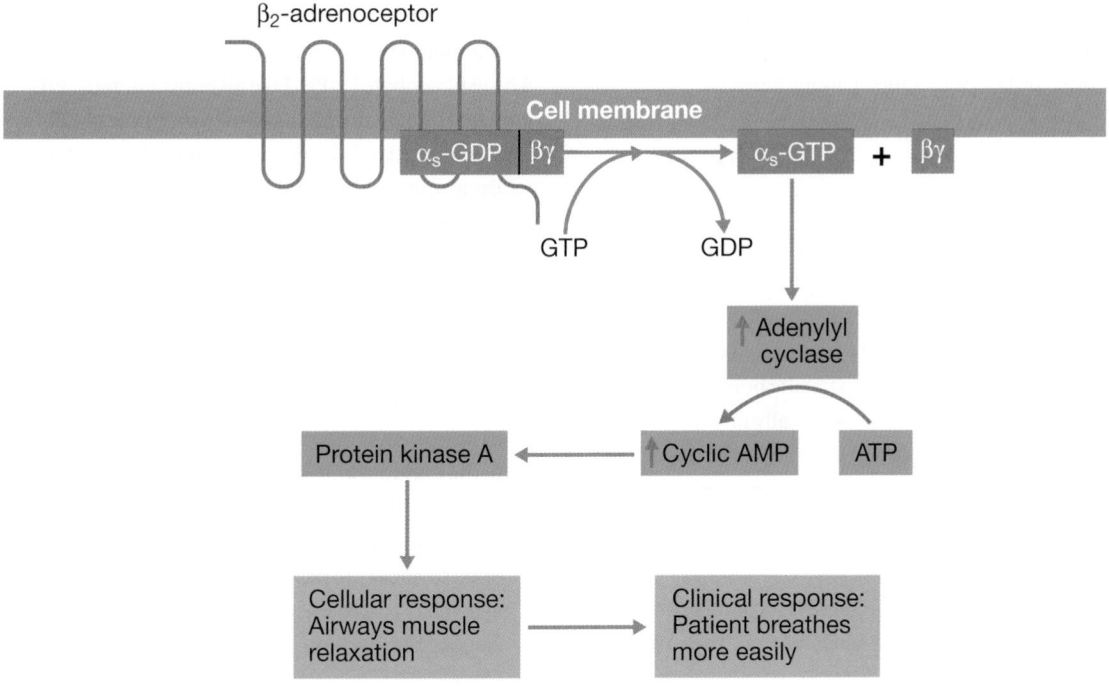

Figure 2.12 Stimulation of β₂-adrenoceptors in bronchiolar smooth muscle increases cyclic AMP synthesis.

The β₂-adrenoceptors are an example of GPCRs coupled through G_s to increases in cyclic AMP levels inside the cell. When the receptor is activated by an agonist it gains affinity for the G_s protein. This coupling causes the release of bound GDP from the α subunit, to be replaced by GTP. This in turn leads to dissociation of the G_s, freeing the $α_s$-GTP subunit which activates adenylyl cyclase, the enzyme responsible for cyclic AMP synthesis. The subsequent increase in intracellular cyclic AMP concentrations activates protein kinase A, which phosphorylates target proteins to bring about the physiological response. In the example here, this response is the relaxation of the smooth muscle cells of the bronchioles.

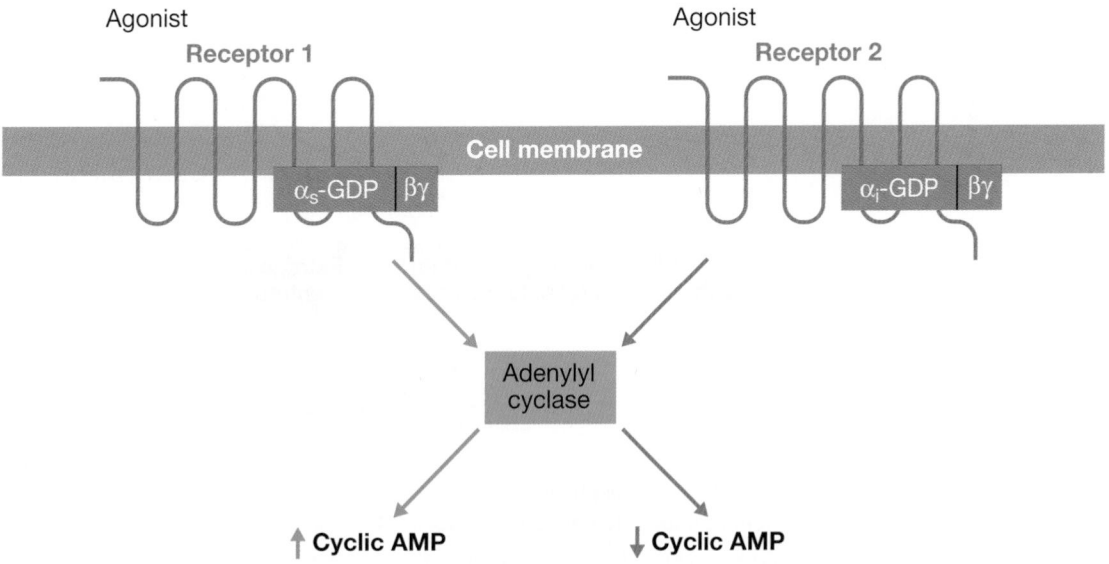

Figure 2.13 Receptors may couple to an inhibition (through G_i) or stimulation (through G_s) of cyclic AMP synthesis.

Note that the scheme shows two different receptors, one of which couples to G_s and one to G_i, and that the increase or decrease in cyclic AMP synthesis is caused by agonists acting at their respective receptors.

synthesis, but also by the use of **phosphodiesterase inhibitors**. This strategy is encountered, for example, when we cover cardiovascular medications in Part 2.

GPCR control of the phospholipase C pathway regulates the function of most cells and tissues

A further subtype of the G protein, G_q, couples receptors to the activation of a phospholipase. Phospholipases are a group of enzymes which split membrane phospholipids into two fragments. Different phospholipases generate different products by acting at specific points on the phospholipid molecule. It is specifically phospholipase C (PLC) that we are interested in here. It is important to gain an understanding of this complex receptor-activated pathway because of its enormous importance for bodily function and drug action.

Following stimulation of G_q-coupled receptors by an agonist, the α_q-GTP subunit activates PLC. The substrate

for this enzyme is the minor component of the phospholipid bilayer, phosphatidylinositol 4,5-bisphosphate (PIP_2). Like all phospholipids, PIP_2 contains both hydrophobic and hydrophilic moieties; the hydrophobic part is buried in the phospholipid bilayer, whilst the phosphorylated sugar (inositol) portion pokes into the cytosol (Figure 2.14). When PIP_2 is cleaved by PLC, two fragments are generated; both are second messengers that influence most aspects of bodily function.

1) The hydrophilic part of the molecule, the sugar with phosphates attached, is inositol 1,4,5-trisphosphate (IP_3). This small molecule diffuses through the cytosol to its protein target, the IP_3 receptors on the membrane of the endoplasmic reticulum, an intracellular store of Ca^{2+}. The IP_3 receptors are examples of ligand-gated ion channels, and when activated by IP_3 binding they open to allow the passage of Ca^{2+} from the store to the cytosol. IP_3 therefore controls **Ca^{2+} levels in the cell**, causing the cytosolic calcium concentration ($[Ca^{2+}]_c$)

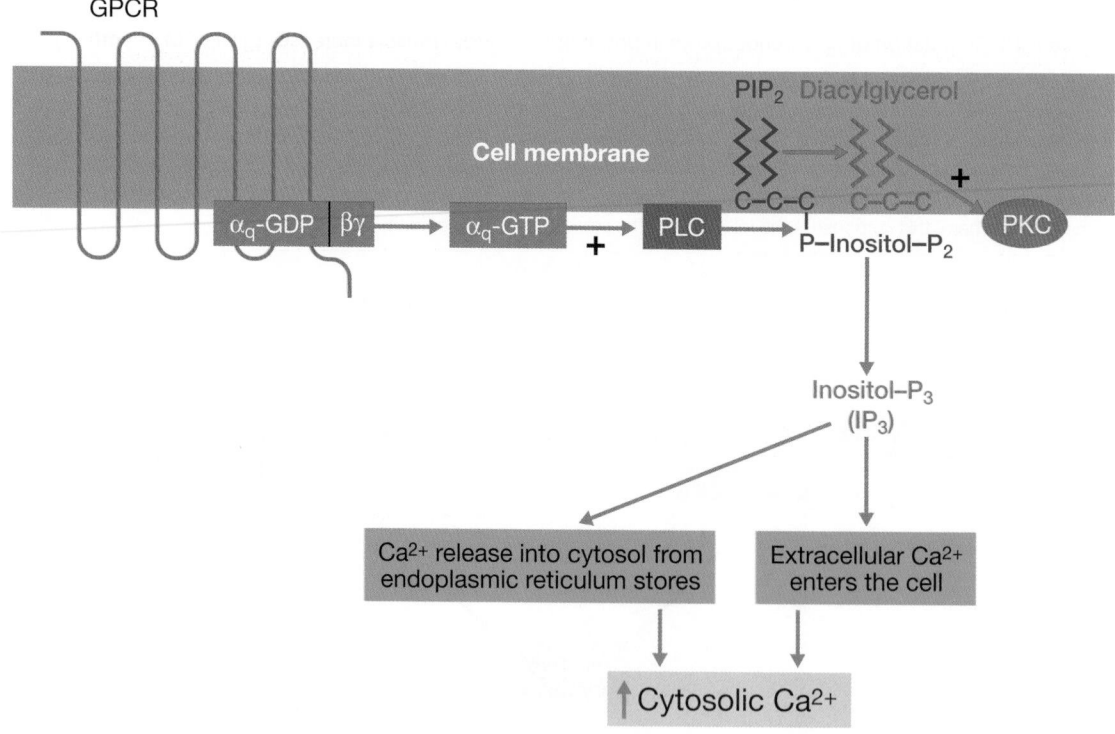

Figure 2.14 Receptor-regulated activation of phospholipase C (PLC) and formation of diacylglycerol and inositol 1,4,5-trisphosphate (IP_3) from its substrate phosphatidylinositol 4,5-bisphosphate (PIP_2).

The GPCR, on binding an agonist, acts through the heterotrimeric protein G_q to activate the enzyme PLC. The substrate of PLC shown in blue is PIP_2. This has a three-carbon glycerol backbone, with fatty acid chains (indicated by the zigzag lines) attached to two of the three glycerol carbons. The third carbon is linked through a phosphate group to an inositol sugar unit which is phosphorylated in two further positions. PLC cleaves this molecule into two fragments such that the three phosphate groups remain attached to the inositol to form IP_3. This molecule is water soluble and diffuses through the cytosol to bring about increases in Ca^{2+} levels. The remaining lipid fragment of PIP_2 is diacylglycerol, which remains in the phospholipid bilayer where it activates the enzyme protein kinase C. GPCR, G protein-coupled receptor; GTP, guanosine-5'-triphosphate.

within the cell to rise from its basal level of around 100 nM in a fast and often highly localized way. Cytosolic Ca^{2+} controls many aspects of cell and tissue function, from muscle contraction and gland secretion, to cell division and cell death.

2) The remaining lipid fraction of PIP_2 is diacylglycerol. This stays in the membrane, from where it acts on protein kinase C (PKC), which migrates from the cytosol to become activated. A large number of PKC subtypes exist with specific cellular distributions. PKC acts to regulate a wide variety of intracellular proteins through phosphorylation, thereby influencing many different aspects of the function of most cells and tissues. The activation of PKC by diacylglycerol is a Ca^{2+}-dependent process, and so the effects of IP_3 and the activation of PKC act in tandem to bring about their biological effects.

2.2.5 Tyrosine kinase receptors: the insulin receptor as an example

The third major class of cell surface receptor to consider is the superfamily of tyrosine kinase receptors (see Figure 2.8). An example is the insulin receptor, a subject

of obvious importance in understanding a number of diseases and their treatment, and in particular the way the body handles glucose and the various forms of diabetes.

In Figure 2.8 we have shown these receptors as two subunits, each crossing the membrane once. Many **growth factor receptors** have this structure. For the **insulin receptor**, however, each of these transmembrane subunits has an additional extracellular subunit attached, as shown in Figure 2.15.

The basic mechanism of all tyrosine kinase receptors is that agonist binding to the extracellular face leads to the phosphorylation of the intracellular domain, which in turn leads to the activation of complex signalling pathways. In the case of insulin this includes not only changes in glucose metabolism and uptake, but also signalling to the nucleus to control gene expression and the cell cycle.

2.2.6 Intracellular receptors

We shall use as our main example here the actions of **corticosteroids**, which are explored in their clinical drug context in Part 3.

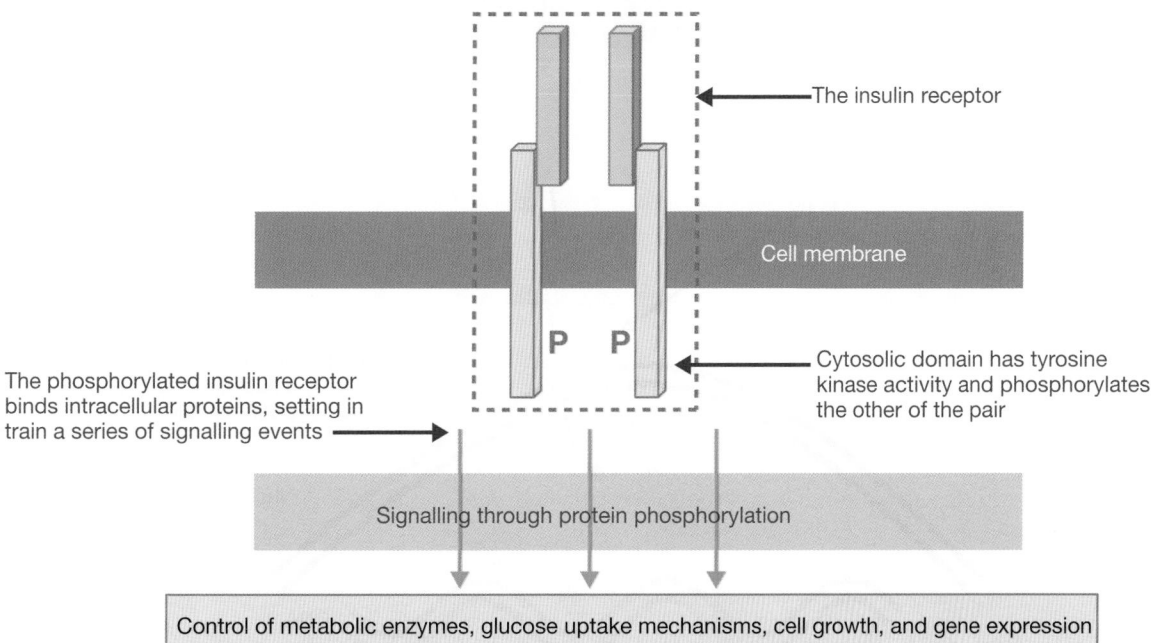

Figure 2.15 The insulin receptor as an example of a tyrosine kinase receptor.

The insulin receptor is composed of the basic tyrosine kinase receptor structure, with two protein subunits each crossing the cell membrane once, but has two additional extracellular subunits. The binding of insulin to the extracellular domain leads to autophosphorylation in the intracellular domain; the kinase activity of each chain phosphorylates the other. As a result the intracellular part of the receptor attracts proteins, which bind to it, and the complex then activates signalling cascades.

Steroids change gene expression

An important property of steroids, both natural ligands and drugs, is that they can enter the cells that they influence. Adrenaline, insulin, and many of the other agonists we shall consider are not lipid soluble, and so cannot cross the cell membrane. To influence the cell they must therefore bind to receptors that are accessible from outside, and as we have already seen in Sections 2.2.2–2.2.4, the receptors must then send signals across the membrane. Steroids, however, are lipid soluble and so pass through the cell membrane into the cell, where they bind to intracellular protein receptors. There are two main classes of these intracellular (or 'nuclear') receptors.

1) Class I receptors are located in the cytosol, in which case the ligand–receptor complex then translocates to the nucleus. The anti-inflammatory corticosteroid drugs central to the treatment of conditions such as rheumatoid arthritis (Chapter 9) and asthma (Chapter 11) act at this type of receptor.

2) Class II receptors are localized to the nucleus, and the ligand–receptor complex forms there.

In both cases, the ligand–receptor complex directly interacts with DNA to modify gene transcription, the exact nature of which depends on the ligand, the receptor, and the cell involved. In the case of the anti-inflammatory corticosteroids that are so important in clinical practice, the result is the reduced expression of genes that cause and promote inflammation and an increase in expression of genes encoding anti-inflammatory proteins (Figure 2.16). It is because of this combined mechanism that anti-inflammatory steroids are so effective.

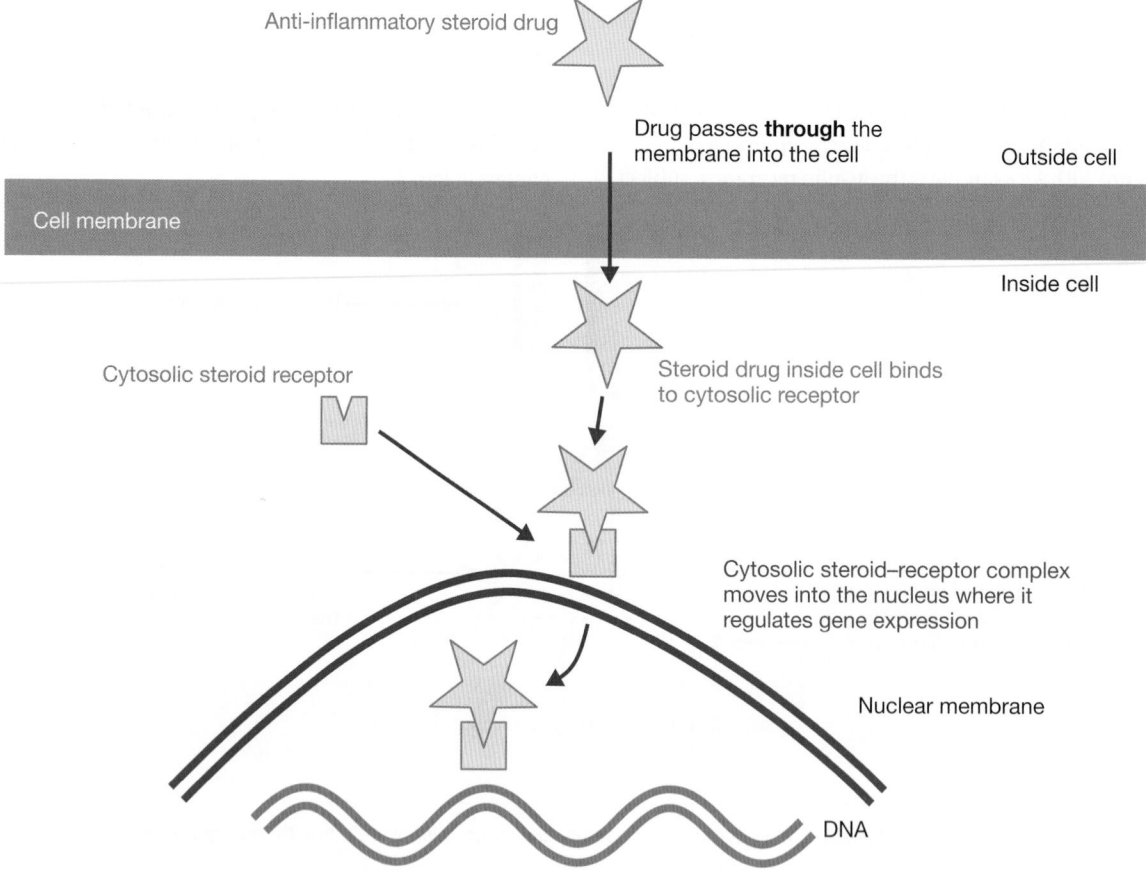

Figure 2.16 Steroid drugs act on intracellular receptors.
The steroid molecule passes straight through the membrane and binds to its receptor inside the cell; this complex enters the nucleus to change gene expression. As the drug is an anti-inflammatory glucocorticoid, gene expression changes in the direction of increased expression of genes for anti-inflammatory proteins (e.g. that for lipocortin), and decreased expression of genes for pro-inflammatory proteins (e.g. inflammatory cytokines).

2.3 Ion channels as drug targets

Ion channels are intrinsic membrane protein complexes that span the cell membrane and, when opened, allow the passage of ions across the otherwise impermeable lipid bilayer. We have encountered one class of ion channel already in Figures 2.8 and 2.9—the ligand-gated ion channel, in which the receptor and the channel protein are one and the same. Ion channels are usually cell surface drug targets.

2.3.1 Voltage-gated channels

These channels are dependent on changes to the potential difference across the cell membrane to determine whether they are open or closed. Muscle cells and nerve cells (excitable cells) have an electric charge across their cell membrane that at rest is negative to about –70 mV inside the cell compared with outside. Some of the ion channels we are interested in are closed under these conditions. If an action potential starts to depolarize the membrane to, say, –40 mV inside, voltage-sensitive Na^+ channels may open, allowing Na^+ into the cell along its concentration gradient. As the membrane becomes even less polarized, moving towards a positive charge inside the cell, voltage-sensitive Ca^{2+} channels (for example, L-type channels on smooth muscle cells) may open, and Ca^{2+} can then flow into the cell (Ca^{2+} is also at a higher concentration outside the cell than in the cytosol). Under some circumstances the voltage-sensitive K^+ channels may open; K^+ will then flow *out* of the cell, as its concentration is higher *inside* than outside the cell. This movement of K^+ will tend to restore the membrane to the resting –70 mV on the inside.

We will encounter all these types of voltage-gated channels later on, as well as drugs that specifically block certain of them, such as amlodipine, an L-type Ca^{2+} channel blocker used in the treatment of hypertension. There are also drugs that open channels, such as nicorandil, which increases the opening of a type of K^+ channel sensitive to intracellular ATP.

Voltage-gated ion channel drugs can be 'use-dependent'

When a voltage-gated Na^+ channel in a nerve cell has opened, allowing Na^+ into the cell and so exciting it, the channel will rapidly close. For a very short time it will enter a state in which it *cannot* be opened—the refractory state. There are some drugs which bind to voltage-gated Na^+ channels in this refractory state. The effect of such drugs is greatest when cells are very active (i.e. producing high frequency action potentials) and so these drugs are referred to as 'use-dependent'. They provide a more sophisticated way of manipulating voltage-sensitive channels than simply blocking them, and such drugs have found clinical use in the treatment of cardiac arrhythmias (Chapter 7) and epilepsy (Chapter 16). The principle of 'use-dependence' is described more fully in Box 16.2.

2.4 Enzymes as drug targets

When an enzyme is a drug target we normally think of intracellular enzymes. We have already noted that this is not always the case, as when the blood plasma enzymes necessary for blood clotting are inhibited by heparins (see Chapter 4).

In the majority of cases therapeutic drugs acting at enzymes cause their inhibition. However, activity through an enzymic step may be *increased* by clinically useful drugs, as when levodopa is used to boost dopamine levels in the brain; in this case the supply of levodopa to the decarboxylase enzyme is increased by its administration as a drug, which is then converted into dopamine (Chapter 17).

2.5 Transporter proteins as drug targets

The simplest examples of this type of drug action are antidepressants which act as inhibitors of the uptake of specific types of neurotransmitter in the brain. The general situation here, with respect to a synapse in the brain, is illustrated in Figure 2.17.

Some of these antidepressants inhibit the uptake of noradrenaline (norepinephrine) and serotonin (5-hydroxytryptamine, 5-HT), for example. When a neurotransmitter is released in the brain, in many cases it is removed by being drawn into local cells, across the cell

28

Chapter 2 How do drugs work? An introduction

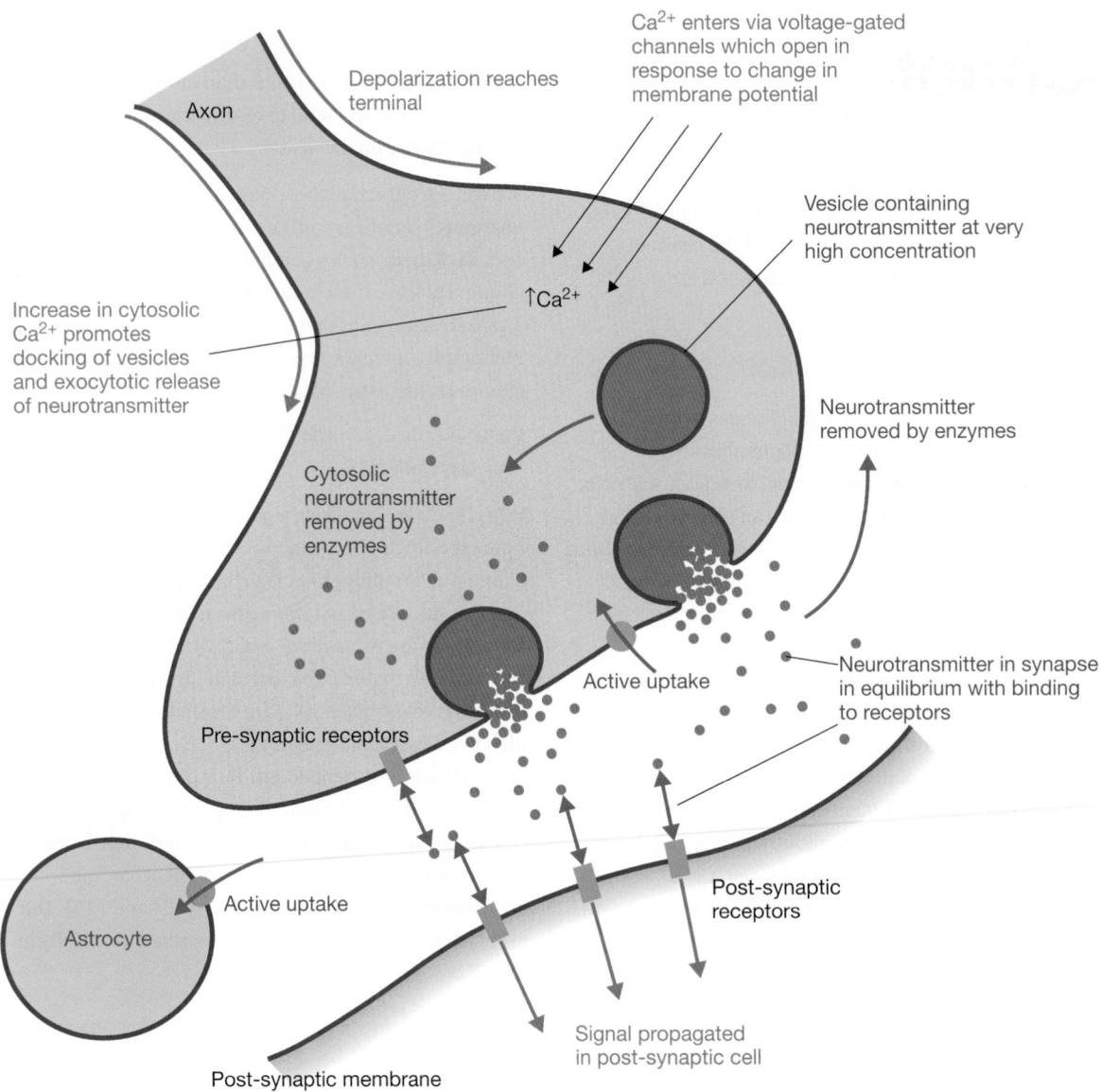

Figure 2.17 The synapse, neurotransmitter, and uptake.

The diagram shows a nerve terminal with neurotransmitter released into the synaptic space. While there, the neurotransmitter molecules can stimulate the receptors (both post-synaptic, mediating neurotransmission, and pre-synaptic, controlling further neurotransmitter release). The neurotransmitter is rapidly removed from the synaptic space; in the case of brain neurotransmitters (e.g. noradrenaline, dopamine, and serotonin) this is largely through active uptake by transporter proteins in the membranes of the nerve terminal or adjacent cells. Drugs that inhibit this reuptake, such as certain antidepressant drugs (see Chapter 19), can be expected to increase the availability of neurotransmitter to stimulate its receptors.

membrane. This is achieved by specific uptake proteins capable of picking up the neurotransmitter and transporting it from the synapse, across the cell membrane, and into the cell, thus terminating its action. Drugs which bind and block these uptake proteins will increase the amount of neurotransmitter in the synapse, thus boosting its activity in the brain. This accounts for the action of some very well-known antidepressant drugs such as fluoxetine and citalopram. Their action is explored more fully in Chapter 19.

Chapter 3
Pharmacokinetics

Useful terms for this topic

Bioavailability: The fraction of the total ingested dose of a drug that gains access to the systemic circulation.

Clearance: Volume of blood cleared of drug per unit time.

Cytochrome P450 (CYP) enzymes: Group of hepatic enzymes that metabolize drugs, converting them to substances that are easier to eliminate.

First-pass metabolism: The metabolism of an orally administered drug as it passes across the intestinal wall and through the liver, before entering the systemic circulation.

Half-life: The time taken for the concentration of drug in the plasma to be halved.

Hepatic extraction ratio: The fraction of drug removed from the plasma by the liver.

Intrinsic clearance: Ability of hepatic enzymes to metabolize a drug.

Pro-drug: An inactive drug that undergoes metabolism (e.g. by the liver) to yield the active compound.

Therapeutic index/window: Comparison of the amount of drug required for a therapeutic effect with the amount that causes toxicity. The narrower this is, the less safe is the drug.

Volume of distribution: Theoretical volume that would contain the total amount of administered drug at the same concentration as that seen in the plasma. A large volume reflects distribution of the drug in tissues around the body (e.g. in fat stores).

Pick up any drug monograph and hidden among information about the dosage, indications, precautions, and side effects will be something about the **pharmacokinetics** of the drug. The term 'pharmacokinetics' quite literally means drug (pharmaco) movement (kinetics), and is the science related to what happens to a drug when it gets into the body. Put simply, it can be thought of as what the body does to the drug. This is in contrast to **pharmacodynamics**, which is concerned with the action of drugs or, in other words, what the drug does to the body. The relationship between pharmacokinetics and pharmacodynamics is outlined in Figure 3.1.

This chapter will review the basics of pharmacokinetics. The study of this topic is a branch of pharmaceutical science in its own right, and this chapter can in no way replace the more comprehensive resources on the subject. A basic understanding of the principles of pharmacokinetics is, however, essential when considering the pharmacology of a drug. After all, pharmacology is literally the science of the interaction of a drug with the body, and the pharmacokinetics of a drug can dictate everything from the route of administration through to how long its effect will last, side effects, and precautions with its use.

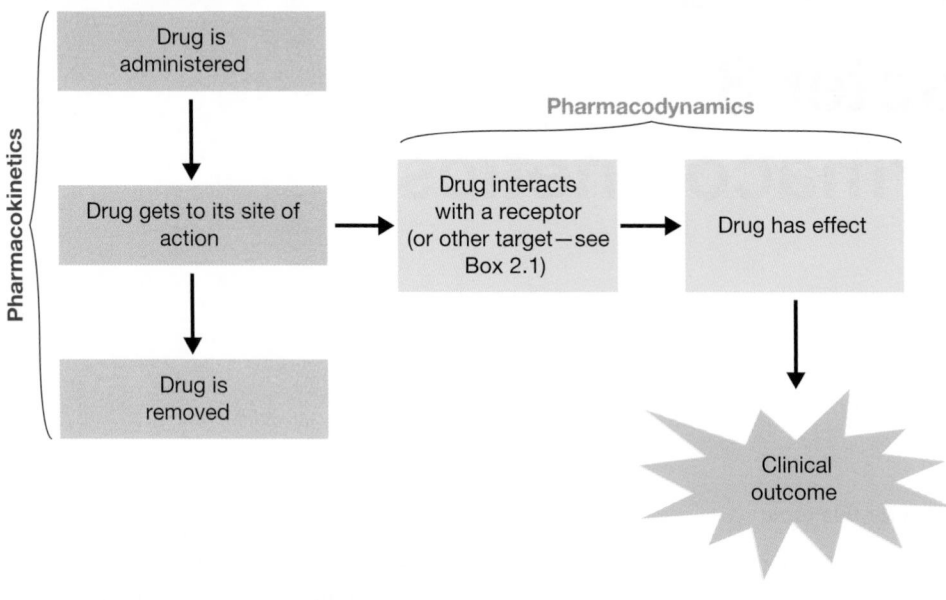

Figure 3.1 Pharmacokinetic aspects of a drug compared with pharmacodynamics.

3.1 The core principles of pharmacokinetics: ADME

When you read about the pharmacokinetics of a drug you will often come across the acronym **ADME**. This stands for:

- **Absorption**
- **Distribution**
- **Metabolism**
- **Elimination.**

These are the four key aspects of the pharmacokinetics of a drug. In order to understand some of the concepts involved we shall work backwards, starting with elimination and finishing with absorption.

3.2 Drug elimination: clearance

The **elimination** of a drug is its irreversible loss from the body. Drugs can be eliminated in their original form (unchanged) or following conversion to other molecules (metabolized). Metabolism occurs primarily in the liver by hepatocytes, but a number of other cells also have the capacity to convert drugs to different forms. The main route for elimination of drugs, either unchanged or as polar metabolites, is via the kidney in the urine. Some drugs are excreted in bile produced by the liver, and then lost from the body in the faeces. Highly volatile substances or gases (e.g. anaesthetics) may be excreted via the lungs. Small amounts of some drugs are lost in secretions such as sweat and milk; the latter route is of obvious significance because of the potential effects on the baby.

The elimination of a drug from the body can be expressed in terms of **clearance**, a fundamental concept of

pharmacokinetics. Clearance is defined as the volume of plasma cleared of the drug per unit time. Conventionally this is presented as l/h or ml/min. Clearance of a drug can be described in terms of routes of elimination (e.g. renal or metabolic clearance), or as the sum of clearance by all routes (total clearance).

As discussed in Chapter 2, for a drug to have an action there must be a critical number of molecules available to interact with its target. The total clearance of a drug is of obvious importance because it determines the dosage rate required to maintain a certain concentration in the plasma (the fluid part of the blood). The relationship between drug concentration and clearance is

$$\text{dosage rate} = \text{plasma concentration} \times \text{clearance}$$

It follows then that if clearance is reduced, the dosage rate must also be decreased to maintain the same plasma concentration. Therefore administering the drug at the same rate in this situation will lead to an increase in plasma concentration. As seen in the example below, this is important to consider when certain health states (e.g. renal disease) or drug interactions can cause clearance rates to go down, resulting in increased plasma levels that could potentially cause toxicity.

> Steven has chronic obstructive pulmonary disease[1] and is admitted to hospital. He is to be given a water-soluble form of theophylline by intravenous infusion. The recommended plasma level for theophylline is 10–20 mg/l. The total clearance in an average adult male of weight 70 kg is approximately 3 l/h. The goal for Steven is the upper plasma level limit of 20 mg/l. To maintain this concentration Steven would need to be given 60 mg/h (20 mg/l × 3 l/h). However, he is a smoker, and this can increase clearance by as much as 50%, because smoking causes the enzymes in the liver which metabolize theophylline to *increase* in activity (more about this later). So his clearance could be as high as 4.5 l/h, in which case he would need 90 mg/h of theophylline to keep the same concentration.

You can see from this example that plasma concentration and clearance are measured in the same unit of volume (in this case litres) which therefore cancels out in the equation. Also, note in the example that the drug is given by intravenous infusion, so all of the drug accesses the bloodstream at a constant rate. A graph of the plasma levels of the drug would look something like Figure 3.2.

As seen in Figure 3.2, initially the drug is being administered faster than it is being cleared, and its concentration in the plasma rises. However, as the drug continues to be given, a plateau is eventually reached

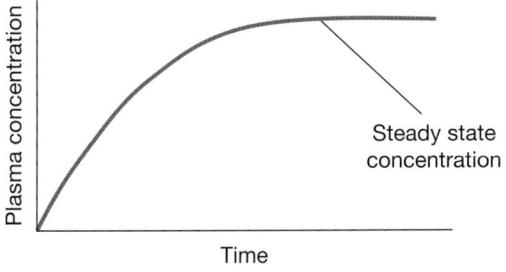

Figure 3.2 Plasma concentration over time for a drug administered by continuous intravenous infusion.

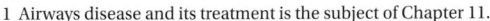

1 Airways disease and its treatment is the subject of Chapter 11.

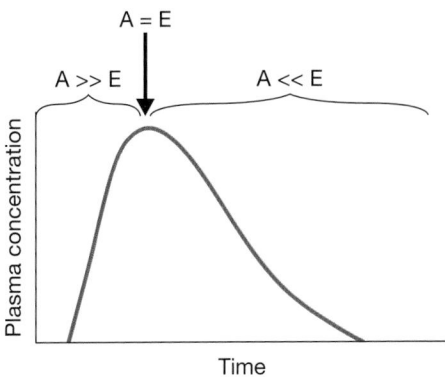

Figure 3.3 Plasma concentration over time for a single dose of drug administered orally.

A, rate of absorption; E, rate of elimination.

where rate of administration is equal to rate of clearance; this is called the steady state concentration.

The situation is quite different when drugs are given orally, as they must first be absorbed into the bloodstream. This absorption may not be complete (see Section 3.5), and is not immediate. Therefore the concentration curve for a dose of an oral medication appears more like that shown in Figure 3.3.

Initially, there is a short delay until the drug starts being absorbed from the small intestine (see Section 3.5). Then its level in the plasma starts to rise, as the rate of absorption is faster than the rate of clearance. The drug reaches its maximal plasma concentration (C_{max}) when the rate of absorption is equal to the rate of elimination. The time at which this occurs is referred to as t_{max}. Plasma concentration of the drug then starts to fall, as the body eliminates the drug faster than it is being absorbed.

3.2.1 Drug elimination by the liver: metabolic clearance

The liver plays a vital role in eliminating foreign molecules, including drugs, from the body through metabolism, which facilitates their elimination. Drugs undergo two kinds of reactions, known as phase I and phase II, which often occur sequentially. Phase I reactions include hydroxylation, oxidation, and dealkylation. The enzymes most often involved in the phase I reactions are members of the **cytochrome P450** family (often abbreviated to CYP or P450). They are located in the smooth endoplasmic reticulum of hepatocytes, the main functional cell type in the liver. The purpose of phase I reactions is to prepare the molecule for subsequent phase

II reactions. The phase I products themselves can be active metabolites, sometimes more active than the parent compound. Phase II reactions include glucuronidation, acetylation, and conjugation, and also take place mainly in the liver although other tissues such as lung, kidney, and intestines can be involved. The phase II reactions usually result in more polar molecules with increased water solubility, aiding their removal by the kidney (see Section 3.2.2). With a few exceptions, for example morphine, the products of the phase II reactions are usually inactive metabolites. For some drugs, hepatic metabolism is a requirement to *activate* the drug, in which case the parent compound is called a pro-drug (e.g. clopidogrel; see Chapter 4).

Hepatic extraction ratio

As blood passes through the liver drug molecules will be presented to hepatocytes for possible metabolic clearance. Many drugs are 'carried' in the blood attached to proteins, the main one being albumin (Figure 3.4). Generally, it is only free (unbound) drug that can be taken up by hepatocytes and metabolized.

The activity of hepatic enzymes to metabolize a drug is known as **intrinsic clearance**. There are therefore three factors that impact on hepatic clearance of drugs: liver blood flow, protein binding, and intrinsic clearance.

If the liver has a low intrinsic clearance of a drug, the rate of hepatic clearance is related to the degree of protein binding and the enzyme activity, and does not depend on liver blood flow. In essence, the liver is so poor at

removing the drug that it doesn't matter how fast or slowly you present the drug to it (i.e. liver blood flow). To visualize this, imagine the liver enzymes are a robotic arm that takes balls off a conveyer belt, and the speed at which the conveyer belt moves is liver blood flow. If the arm is very slow at removing the balls, say only taking one off every hour, it doesn't matter how slow or fast the conveyer belt moves, because it still only takes off very few!

Conversely, if the liver has high levels of enzyme activity for a drug, the main determinant of hepatic clearance is liver blood flow. Using the example above, the robotic arm is so efficient that it could potentially remove the balls faster than the conveyer belt can carry them. Therefore, how many are removed will depend on the speed at which they are presented.

The ratio of the hepatic clearance of a drug to the blood flow through the liver is termed the **hepatic extraction ratio**. This can range from 0 (no drug removed by the liver) to 1 (all of the drug is removed on one pass through the liver). For example, if a drug has a hepatic extraction ratio of 0.7, it means that 70% of the drug is removed each time the blood passes through the liver. Given that the average hepatic blood flow is 1.5 l/h, this would mean that the hepatic clearance would be approximately 1 l/h (i.e. $0.7 \times 1.5 = 1.05$). Knowing whether the liver has high or low capacity for metabolizing a drug helps predict which factors will impact on its clearance, as we can see in this example.

Margaret is taking warfarin, because of a long history of repeated deep vein thromboses,[2] and propranolol for anxiety.[3] She develops a chest infection and her GP decides to prescribe a macrolide antibiotic,[4] erythromycin. He checks to see if this could cause any problems, and finds that erythromycin can increase the effect of warfarin but has little effect on propranolol, even though both are metabolized by the liver. The difference is that warfarin has low clearance by the liver (hepatic extraction ratio <0.3), whereas that of propranolol is high (hepatic extraction ratio ~0.7). The interaction with warfarin occurs because erythromycin is an inhibitor of hepatic enzymes (CYP450). This reduces the clearance of warfarin, thereby increasing its levels and effectiveness. In contrast, because the liver has a much greater capacity to metabolize propranolol, its clearance from the plasma is hardly affected when some of the enzymes are blocked by erythromycin.

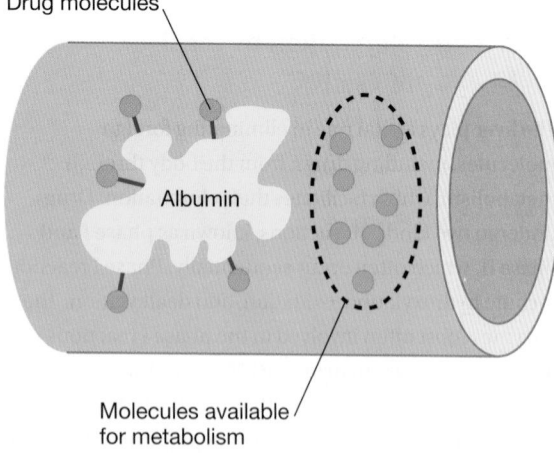

Drug molecules

Albumin

Molecules available for metabolism

Figure 3.4 Example of drug binding to albumin.

2 Chapter 4.
3 Chapter 19.
4 Chapter 22.

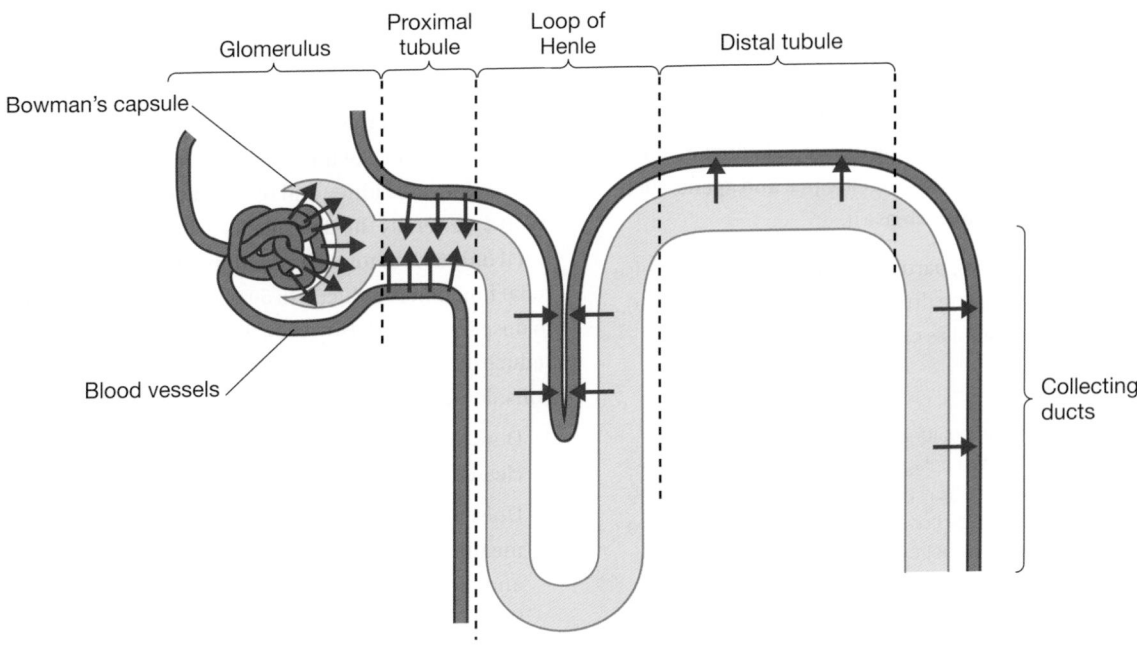

Figure 3.5 Major elements of the kidney.
The arrows indicate the directions in which drugs can travel, both into the filtrate from the plasma (filtration and secretion), and out of the filtrate and back into the plasma through reabsorption.

3.2.2 Elimination by the kidney

The kidney is a complex organ and is the major site of drug elimination. The key parts of the nephron, the functional unit of the kidney, are outlined in Figure 3.5.

In the kidney, drugs can undergo three processes: **filtration**, **secretion**, or **reabsorption**. The kidney filters drugs and other substances through the glomerulus (an intertwined mass of semipermeable blood vessels that sits inside the Bowman's capsule) and clears approximately 10% of the plasma as it passes through at a rate of about 1200 ml/min. Thus the glomerular filtration rate is about 120 ml/min. The process of filtration is passive and only unbound drugs are filtered.

The nephron also has several active transport systems that are located in the proximal tubule. The two main systems affect acidic drugs (e.g. penicillin) and basic drugs (e.g. procainamide). These transporters 'pump' drugs from the bloodstream across the walls of the proximal tubule into the filtrate. Drugs that compete for these **secretion** methods can lead to decreased clearance of other drugs, and so to potential toxicity. This competition is exploited therapeutically when

probenecid is given with penicillins. Probenecid slows the elimination of penicillin by competing for the tubular secretion mechanism, thereby prolonging its effects. Unlike glomerular filtration, these secretory transport systems can clear drugs bound to plasma proteins.

As the glomerular filtrate passes along the nephron most components, including 99% of the water, are reabsorbed from, in turn, the proximal tubule, the loop of Henle, the distal tubule, and the collecting ducts. Only 1–2 ml of the original 120 ml filtered from the plasma each minute is eventually excreted as urine. Thus the concentration of drugs that are only filtered increases approximately 100-fold along the length of the nephron (e.g. 1 mg of drug present in the 120 ml of plasma originally filtered, would be concentrated in the final 1–2 ml lost as urine). This increase in concentration encourages passive reabsorption, which is influenced by two factors.

1. Filtration volume. Drinking large volumes of water increases filtration, and decreases reabsorption of water from the nephron to produce urine that is more dilute. This will decrease the concentration of drugs in the urine, thereby decreasing their reabsorption which is dependent on concentration gradient.

2. Only un-ionized (non-charged) molecules can pass through membranes to be reabsorbed. However, drugs that are weak acids or weak bases can change their state of ionization depending on the pH of the urine. This can be modified using urinary alkalinizers such as sodium bicarbonate to increase pH, and agents such as ascorbic acid to decrease it.

These two influences, particularly urinary pH, can cause interactions with some drugs (increasing their toxicity), but can also be useful as can be seen in the following example:

> As part of his treatment for lymphoma, Simon is given methotrexate, a folate antagonist anticancer drug.[5] While he is receiving the drug, he is given plenty of fluid and a urinary alkalinizer, sodium bicarbonate. This is done to enhance the renal clearance of methotrexate by first increasing its dilution in the urine, making it less likely to be reabsorbed. Second, methotrexate is a weak acid (pKa = 4.3) and therefore is ionized in alkaline urine, reducing its ability to cross membranes. This interaction is used to reduce the toxicity of methotrexate to the kidneys by increasing its removal.

Why is renal clearance important?

Understanding the factors that influence renal excretion helps predict drug interactions (as described above) as well as the effect of disease states, most notably renal dysfunction. Irrespective of whether a drug is actively secreted or passively reabsorbed, the most important determinant of renal elimination is filtration. We measure renal (or glomerular) filtration rate using **clearance of creatinine**, a waste product of the breakdown of creatine phosphate in the muscle. It is primarily filtered, with very little secretion and no reabsorption, and therefore its rate of clearance gives an approximation of glomerular filtration rate. Using serum creatinine levels, and adjusting for age, weight, and gender, it is possible to calculate this rate using a formula developed by Cockcroft and Gault in 1976 (often referred to as the 'Cockcroft–Gault equation'):

$$\text{creatine clearance} = \frac{(140 - \text{age}) \times (\text{weight in kg})}{814 \times \text{serum creatinine(mmol/l)}}$$
$$[\times 0.85 \text{ for females}]$$

As a rule, for most drugs adjustment for reduced renal filtration is only required if creatinine clearance has

decreased by 50% or more (i.e. <60 ml/min). If required, the dosage adjustment is usually proportional to the degree of reduction in renal clearance, but it must also take into account the contribution of renal clearance to the total clearance of the drug. If a drug is entirely removed by the kidney and renal function is decreased by 50%, generally the dose needs to be reduced by 50%. But if only 50% of total elimination is by the kidneys, and renal function is reduced to 50%, only a 25% reduction in dose is required. However, when deciding whether to reduce doses in renal failure two things must be considered.

1. Does the drug have active metabolites that are also cleared by the kidneys?

2. Does the drug have a low **therapeutic index**, meaning that the difference between toxic levels and therapeutic levels is small? In this case, the need for dose reduction in renal failure may be more critical.

3.2.3 Protein binding

We have seen that with both renal filtration and hepatic clearance, only free (or unbound) drug is removed from the plasma. In addition, only free drug is available to interact with receptors to give a pharmacological effect. As mentioned above, drugs can be bound to proteins in the plasma, including albumin, α_1-acid glycoprotein, and lipoproteins. The most abundant plasma protein is albumin, which binds and carries many endogenous substances such as bilirubin and hormones, and which can also bind drugs. α_1-acid glycoprotein is an acute phase protein that increases in concentration in response to systemic tissue injury and inflammation, and contains a single binding site. Lipoproteins are macromolecular complexes of lipids, cholesterol, and proteins (see Chapter 6) to which drugs can bind, and be carried in the plasma.

Protein binding is similar to competitive receptor binding (see Chapter 2) in that free and bound drugs exist in equilibrium:

$$\text{free drug} + \text{protein} \rightleftarrows \text{drug–protein complex}$$

The degree of protein binding is determined by the physicochemical properties of the drug and its affinity for the protein, the concentration of free drug, and the amount of protein available. Examples of drugs which

---

5 Cancer drug therapy is discussed in Chapter 23.

are highly protein bound are warfarin, propranolol, phenytoin, and diazepam. The degree of protein binding can change due to displacement (another drug or endogenous molecule 'pushing' the bound molecule off the carrier) or reduced levels of proteins (e.g. in hepatic failure, as albumin is synthesized in the liver).

As you would expect, changes in protein binding primarily affect drugs that are highly protein bound. A decrease in protein binding initially leads to a rise in the concentration of free drug. However, this unbound drug can now be eliminated; more drug is cleared, and the concentration of free drug returns to the starting level. Overall, though, the *total* concentration of drug in the plasma will go down, as more has been eliminated. The net effect is a reduction in total drug concentration, with little change in the level which is not bound to protein (Figure 3.6).

Because the levels of free drug remain largely unaltered, and it is this that exerts the pharmacological effect, changes in protein binding do not usually alter the

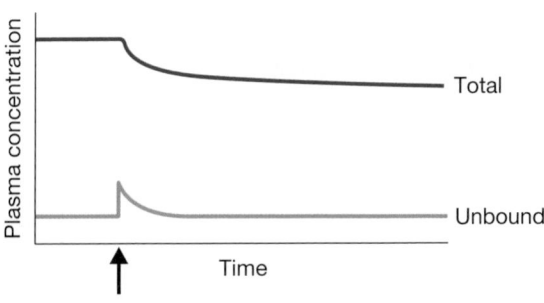

Figure 3.6 Comparison of total and unbound drug concentrations following protein displacement (at time indicated by the arrow).

effect of the drug. It is, however, an important consideration when interpreting plasma levels during therapeutic drug monitoring, which are often given as the total level of drug in the plasma. (So, reduced total plasma level of the drug would usually be a sign to increase its dose. But if protein binding is also reduced, the free drug level, and therefore the therapeutic effectiveness, may be unchanged.)

3.3 Volume of distribution

The second fundamental concept of pharmacokinetics is the **volume of distribution** (V_d), which is defined as the volume that would contain the total body content of the administered drug at a concentration equal to that present in the plasma. As such, it is a virtual volume, usually referred to as the apparent volume of distribution. V_d reflects the extent to which the drug distributes into tissues, and binds to proteins and other structures in the body. The formula to determine V_d is

$$V_d = \frac{\text{total amount in the body}}{\text{concentration in blood/plasma}}$$

If a drug is highly distributed/bound to structures outside the plasma, the V_d is large because the free concentration in plasma will be small (Box 3.1). Conversely, if tissue binding is very low, V_d approximates plasma volume (~5 l). The degree of binding is determined by the physicochemical properties of the drug, including the size of the molecule, its solubility, and the state of ionization.

Examples of V_d for some drugs are given in Table 3.1. Highly lipid-soluble drugs like imipramine and chloroquine have a large V_d, reflecting their propensity to partition into fat stores around the body.

3.3.1 When is knowing V_d helpful?

The V_d is used to calculate the loading dose of a drug—a higher than normal dose used to rapidly achieve steady state levels of drug (see Figure 3.1). In the example given above for Steven, it took some time for theophylline, given by continuous infusion, to reach steady state levels (plateau concentration). Knowing the V_d and concentration of drug required, the equation above can be rearranged to calculate the loading dose.

To get the concentration of theophylline in Steven's plasma rapidly to the desired level (20 mg/l), we can calculate the loading dose as V_d × concentration required. For Steven this would be 30 l × 20 mg/l = 600 mg.

Box 3.1
Volume of distribution

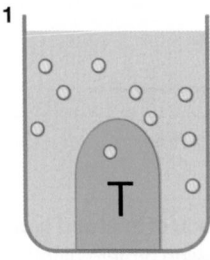 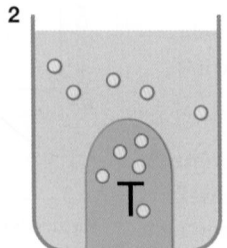 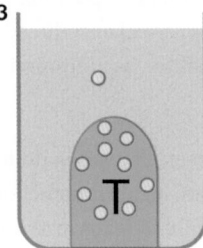

Figure a Volume of distribution.

In Figure a the grey liquid inside the beakers represents plasma and the yellow mass represents tissues (T). For simplicity, let us assume that each beaker contains one litre of liquid. Imagine we have added 10 mg of drug (one red dot represents 1 mg) to each beaker.

$$V_d = \frac{\text{total amount in the body}}{\text{concentration in blood/plasma}}$$

1. In beaker 1, there is very little binding with only 1 mg of drug attached to tissue. The concentration of free drug in the plasma is 9 mg/l and so V_d is 10 mg/9 mg/l = 1.11 l. It can therefore be seen that if binding is very low, V_d approximates the total volume. For a drug in the body V_d would approximate plasma volume (~5 l).

2. In beaker 2 there is modest tissue binding with half of the drug bound. The concentration of free drug in the liquid is 5 mg/l, and V_d is 10 mg/5 mg/l = 2 l.

3. In beaker 3, binding is very high with 9 mg of drug attached to tissue. The concentration of free drug in the liquid is 1 mg/l. Thus V_d is 10 mg/1 mg/l = 10 l (i.e. much greater than the total volume).

Table 3.1 Apparent volumes of distribution for some common drugs

Drug	Apparent V_d (l)
Warfarin*	10
Theophylline	30
Diazepam	80
Imipramine	>1000
Chloroquine	>7000

*V_d for total warfarin (both free and bound to plasma proteins)

3.4 Half-life of a drug

The **plasma half-life** of a drug is the time it takes for its concentration to be halved. After administering a single bolus injection of a drug, plasma levels decrease over time as shown in Figure 3.7. The half-life of the hypothetical drug depicted is 2 hours; it takes this length of time for the plasma concentration to drop from 100 mg/l to 50 mg/l, and to halve again to 25 mg/l.

The half-life ($t_{1/2}$) is related to the two key parameters already discussed, V_d and clearance, by the following formula:

$$t_{1/2} = \frac{0.693 \times V_d}{\text{clearance}}$$

This tells us that changes in V_d and clearance have opposite effects on half-life. If V_d decreases (e.g. if binding to tissues changes), the half-life of the drug also decreases because more is now available for elimination. Conversely, if the rate of clearance of a drug decreases (e.g. in renal or hepatic disease), its half-life will increase.

3.4.1 Why is knowing the half-life of a drug useful?

Firstly, as seen in Figure 3.7, the half-life enables us to predict how drug levels will fall. As there is usually a minimum concentration of a drug required in the plasma to give an effect, this information helps predict the duration of action after a single dose of drug. Using the example in Figure 3.7, and setting the minimum effective concentration at 20 mg/l, a single dose of the drug will be ineffective after just over 4 hours. Because the decline in plasma levels is exponential, and not linear, doubling the dose does not double the duration of action. In Figure 3.7, if twice the dose was administered, giving an initial concentration of 200 mg/l, plasma levels would drop below 20 mg/l after just over 6 hours, and not 8 hours.

Secondly, the half-life helps to determine fluctuations in plasma levels of drug between dosing. This is illustrated taking the example of theophylline again which has a plasma half-life of approximately 4 hours, and a low therapeutic index; levels above 20 mg/l can cause toxicity (e.g. cardiac arrhythmias and neurological side effects), whilst at levels below 10 mg/l it is often ineffective. Figure 3.8 shows two dosing regimens for theophylline in a 20 kg child. In both, a total of 600 mg is given in a 24 hour period. Administering 300 mg every 12 hours leads to a peak plasma concentration of about 35 mg/l, and a trough (lowest) level of about 4.5 mg/l. The drug is only within the therapeutic range (10–20 mg/l) for about 4 hours. Alternatively, if 100 mg of theophylline is given every 4 hours, levels remain within the therapeutic range for the entire period.

For most drugs with half-lives of up to 24 hours, giving doses every half-life is appropriate. However, if a drug has a very short half-life, dosing will be so frequent that patients may find it difficult to keep taking the medicine, leading to non-compliance. Sustained-release preparations which release the drug more slowly over time provide a solution in this situation.

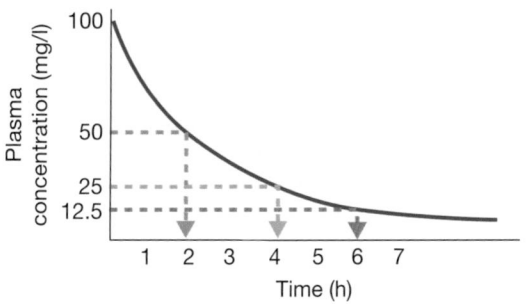

Figure 3.7 Plasma concentration over time for a hypothetical drug with half-life of 2 h.

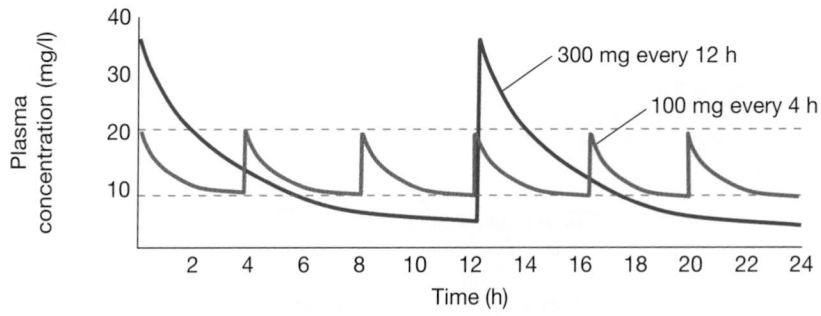

Figure 3.8 Plasma concentration over time with two dosing regimens for theophylline in a 20 kg child.

Adapted from Birkett DJ. Half-life. *Australian Prescriber* 1988; 11(3): 57–9. Copyright NPS MedicineWise.

The third aspect of drug dosing that is determined by the half-life, is the time to reach steady state (see Figure 3.2). With chronic oral dosing, or continuous intravenous infusion, it takes about five half-lives to reach steady state. This helps to determine how long it will take to get to a therapeutic level.

> Julia is rushed into the emergency department with an episode of status epilepticus,[6] a very severe and potentially life-threatening form of epilepsy. One of the drugs used to treat it is phenytoin, which has a half-life of about 24 hours. To avoid delay in reaching the steady state level, the emergency physician gives her a loading dose (a higher than normal dose) of the drug to rapidly achieve therapeutic levels. Once under control, Julia's epilepsy can be maintained with once-daily dosing of phenytoin.

3.5 Absorption and bioavailability

Drugs are given by a variety of routes for a systemic effect, including parenterally (by injection), sublingually, topically, and rectally. The vast majority, though, are given orally. Once swallowed, the tablet or capsule has to disintegrate and/or dissolve; this normally takes place in the stomach. The drug then passes into the small intestine from where it is usually absorbed. This involves crossing the epithelial cell wall of the intestine to be carried via the hepatic portal vein to the liver, from where it enters the systemic circulation. The process of

absorption is influenced by many factors, as outlined in Figure 3.9.

Following absorption, the drug is exposed to possible hepatic metabolism. If the extraction ratio of a drug is very high, little or no drug will be present in the blood which leaves the liver to enter the general circulation. In this case the drug is said to have a high first-pass metabolism (or, that there is a high first-pass effect). The **bioavailability** of such a drug is low; this term denotes

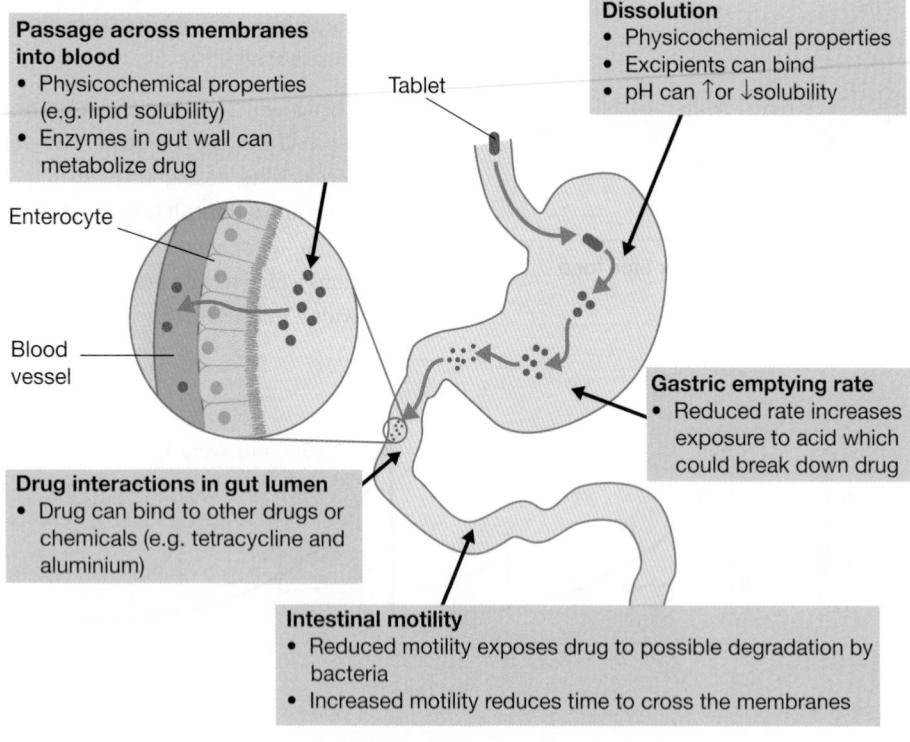

Figure 3.9 Factors influencing the absorption of a drug from a tablet.

6 The subject of epilepsy is introduced in Chapter 16.

the fraction of the total ingested dose of a drug that gains access to the systemic circulation. Drugs with high first-pass metabolism include verapamil, propranolol, and lidocaine. For some drugs, such as glyceryl trinitrate (GTN), a vasodilator used for angina (see Chapter 7) and buprenorphine, an opioid analgesic (see Chapter 20), the hepatic extraction ratio is so high that oral bioavailability is nearly zero. This means that alternative routes of administration must be used. Both drugs are available as topical patches for absorption through the skin. The first-pass effect can also be avoided by sublingual (under the tongue) administration, so that the drug enters the systemic circulation without first passing through the liver. Drugs are sometimes given rectally to avoid first-pass effects. It should, however, be noted that the blood supply from the upper part of the rectum does drain into the liver, and drug absorbed here will therefore be subject to first-pass effects.

As discussed earlier, for drugs with high hepatic extraction ratios, changes in enzyme activity have little effect on systemic clearance. They can, though, have a dramatic effect on its bioavailability. For example, if a drug has an extraction ratio of 90% (0.9) which goes down to 85% (0.85) because of enzyme inhibition, the bioavailability increases from 10% to 15%, a relative increase of 50%.

 ## Key references and suggested reading

Birkett DJ. *Pharmacokinetics Made Easy* (2nd edn). Sydney: McGraw-Hill, 2010.